age 11

To: Mirai.H
from: Aontie Sue

ABOUT BLOODY TIME

THE MENSTRUAL REVOLUTION WE HAVE TO HAVE

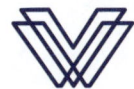

First published in 2019 by the Victorian Women's Trust and its harm prevention entity, The Dugdale Trust for Women & Girls, Level 9/313 La Trobe Street, Melbourne, Victoria 3000, Australia.

Copyright © The Dugdale Trust for Women & Girls, 2019

All rights reserved. Without limiting the rights under copyright above, no part of this publication shall be reproduced, stored in or introduced into a retrieval system, or transmitted in any form or by any means (electronic, mechanical, photocopying, recording or otherwise), without the prior permission of both the copyright owner and the publisher of this book.

Front Cover: Alice Lindstrom

Other images: Lucy Fahey and Michelle Pereira

Design and layout: Aimee Carruthers

Karen Pickering photo: Laura Du Vé

Printed in Melbourne, Australia by The Print Department

Enquiries: women@vwt.org.au

ISBN: 978-0-9873906-7-7

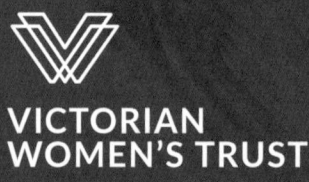

We recognise the Australian Aboriginal and Torres Strait Islander Peoples of this nation as the traditional custodians of this land and its waterways. We acknowledge the privilege of conducting our work on these lands, where sovereignty was never ceded, and we pay our deepest respects to ancestors and Elders. We especially want to pay tribute to the might and resilience of Indigenous women, who have endured and persisted in the face of unimaginable difficulty. We hope that our work helps to ensure dignity and empowerment for the girls and women of the First Nations Peoples of Australia, who face very different challenges in the same society, as part of our commitment to all Australian women and girls.

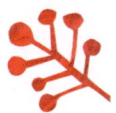

CONTENTS

9
Preface

11
Authors' Note

14
Foreword

18
Introduction

22
Our Data

46
The Biological Integrity of Menstruation

88
A Pervasive Menstrual Taboo

142
Dismantling the Menstrual Taboo

157
Acknowledgements

160
Appendices

202
References and Notes

PREFACE

Preface

In March 2012 a small group of us, seasoned menstrual educators, found ourselves at the same table early one morning in a kitchen at the very first Seven Sisters Festival, held in the country near Shepparton in Victoria; each of us well aware of what it meant to be a menstrual educator in a culture which was deeply and negatively inclined about the word menstruation and everything that went with it. We knew it was time to work together. With the powerful network support of Bindy Gross, we found ourselves with Mary Crooks and Duré Dara at the Victorian Women's Trust. We all felt such a deep excitement – could there be a productive meeting of minds?

Each of us, Jane Hardwicke Collings, Jane Bennett, Lara Owen and myself had over many years visualised a world which framed menstruation as a blessing, an engaged and recognised resource that could actually bring enjoyment to the life lived within a woman's body. We voiced this vision, and in the process, outlined our dream of establishing an institute which could deliver positive and effective menstrual training and education. Having listened intently, Mary leaned forward and said, quietly, 'We can do better than that surely.' Goosebumps. From that moment, with Mary's guidance and the support of Trust staff, we began an epic adventure of making real a bold and ambitious social change agenda which we believed would improve the lives of women and girls in lasting ways.

The book you hold now is the culmination of seven years of gestation and work. In 2015 feminist writer and advocate Karen Pickering joined with Jane Bennett to form a new writing team. Collectively, we've excavated our own practice wisdom and that of others in the field and relished the stories and insights of the several thousand women and girls who participated and gave voice to their lived experience of menstruation in the research phase. We believe that now we offer a framework that can change the way women view the natural power of their own bodies and transform the taboo of menstrual shame into a productive and powerful force to change both our private and shared worlds for the better.

Let the revolution begin!

Katherine Cunningham, January 2019

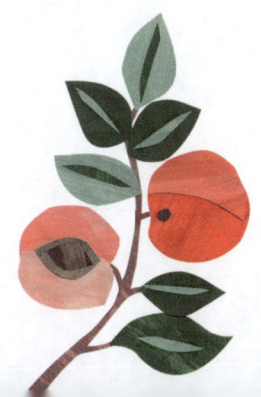

Authors' Note

This book is built on the archive collected during initial work commissioned by The Victorian Women's Trust to collect and gauge the attitudes of women in the community regarding menarche, menstruation and menopause (at the time known as The Waratah Project). We were privileged to hear the thoughts of thousands of women in over fifty countries, but the bulk of responses came from within Australia. You can read about the methodology in the appendices, including how we captured the data.

It was a huge undertaking and revealed clear trends in how women and girls view their menstrual cycle, which we'll demonstrate with close analysis in these pages, but the study could only ask certain questions and investigate a very specific set of attitudes. The sample was complex and diverse, but it was beyond the scope of the research to determine the race, ethnicity, ability and sexuality of every respondent. That said, many of the responses reference these identity markers and wherever possible we include them to give a broader picture of women's experience. In the future, there will be specialised studies and resources on menstruation and menopause that focus especially on the contemporary experience of queer women, disabled women, Indigenous women, Muslim women, migrant and refugee women, gender non-conforming (GNC) people, trans men and other marginalised groups. We very much hope that our generalist approach opens up a space to begin these conversations and that our work can be built on, expanded, critiqued and continued.

We're currently living through an extraordinary time in terms of public understanding of the fluidity of gender and we want to honour and acknowledge the work done by trans and gender non-conforming activists who have held space within progressive movements, for the betterment of all.

We want to be unequivocal in our assertion that trans women are women and that GNC people are challenging our traditional binary notions of gender in powerful and courageous ways. So, a book about menstruation, focusing as it does on the physiological function of (cis) women's bodies is a fraught idea and one that we have grappled with and examined from many different angles. But we always come back to the same place – that if the overwhelming majority of women experience menstruation as a source of shame and stigma and pain, and that patriarchy has prevented them from connecting with the truth that it shouldn't be this way, then we have a responsibility to find a way to have this conversation.

ABOUT BLOODY TIME

Misogyny is material and is often located in bodies. The particular kinds of bodily oppression that cis women face is real and profound, and speaking this truth should take nothing away from acknowledging the very real oppression of trans and GNC people's bodies. There is an important discussion to be had about women whose bodies cannot menstruate, about men who do menstruate, and about people who experience menstruation from the perspective of identifying as neither binary gender, and we hope a book like that comes into existence – written by trans and GNC authors – for the sake of people who need to read it, and for people like us, in the field, who would see it as necessary and significant. This is not that book. Our focus is women who menstruate and how the political category of womanhood is underpinned, undermined and affected by this function of their bodies.[i]

In pursuing these questions, we have used terminology inherited from the medical and scientific communities and aimed to be as precise and consistent as possible. Obviously, there are great critiques to be mounted as to the etymology and origins of many of these words, but it's outside our power to change the word vagina to something less sheath-related, for instance. So please proceed knowing that we understand some of this language may be confronting or frustrating, or in some cases even triggering, for some readers. When we mean vulva, we say vulva, and so on, but designations like 'female reproductive system', 'secondary sexual characteristics', 'sex organs' and 'menses' are also used. Exactitude and uniformity have been our constant goals and we felt this was the best way to increase understanding and knowledge, the better for any reader to go forth and challenge the medical and scientific establishments on their nomenclature, as surely many will agree is long overdue.

Likewise, we want to take this opportunity to acknowledge that much of what is discussed herein may be personal, emotional, and even fraught, for some, particularly when we cover areas like foetal development and survival, sex and sexual relationships, partners and parental responsibilities, and events (like abuse, harassment and other types of interpersonal violence) that have caused distress, humiliation and self-reproach. Please accept this broad content warning that we do mention difficult topics at times and that we have taken as much care as possible to introduce and examine them sensitively.

Something else we refer to in the book, that requires a small usage note of its own, and that is use of the pill and the Pill. The latter refers to all types of hormonal contraception including birth control pills, implants, IUDs, patches and injections. This is partly political and partly stylistic; these products are often differentiated as commercial products but as they contain minor variations of the same one or two drugs in combination (synthetic versions of oestrogen and progesterone) we treat them as the same, or in the same category at least. There are times in the book where we specify a particular delivery method but otherwise you can assume that when we capitalise the Pill it includes them all.

AUTHORS' NOTE

Women and girls everywhere stand to benefit when we pull back the veil of secrecy around menstruation and menopause, and as with most issues of women's rights, positive change will benefit all people in all communities. We are proud and privileged to present the findings of this study and have taken our role as the keepers of these records seriously. The women who took part did so in the belief that sharing their vulnerable moments, deepest fears and dearest hopes would help other women, and we wanted to do justice to that brave impulse: we thank you and we salute you.

Finally, we wish to extend our sincere thanks and deep gratitude to everyone at the Victorian Women's Trust, who have provided support and enthusiasm for this project. We could not have asked for a more encouraging and accommodating environment, and we especially want to acknowledge the collaboration and engagement of Mary Crooks. Mary has been an important contributor, thought leader and true champion of this work, and we have both felt deeply moved by the trust and belief she has shown in us, not to mention the invigorating intellectual debate.

There are a great many other individuals and organisations that have shown interest, engagement and support for this work – without whose expertise and dedication this project would not have come to fruition – and while we haven't listed them all, we offer our genuine gratitude.

We also want to recognise the contribution of our families and thank them for the love, care and nourishment they provided in helping us give our best to this project.

Karen and Jane

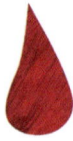
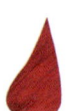

Foreword

Sometime in the middle of the night, shortly after I turned twelve, my period started for the very first time. I sensed something was different when I woke up, and soon discovered what had happened when I went to the bathroom and saw pinkish liquid smeared across scrunched up toilet paper.

Reader, I was thrilled. Finally, the thing that I had been anticipating for so long had happened. I had arrived.

I had been waiting for my period for so long. There were two other bleeders in the house already, my sister and mother, and I was desperate to join their ranks. It seemed to me that menstruation delivered the key to some kind of secret society. I knew about the scientific nature of it, but there was a difference between knowing and knowing. I already felt wise beyond my years, but this surely confirmed it.

(Narrator: She wasn't, and it didn't.)

In the months preceding the start of my first menses, I daydreamed about what I would do when I received its gift. I had pored over copies of *Dolly*, *Girlfriend* and *Just Seventeen*, and I was aware of a reticence among other adolescents to a) embrace menstruation and b) tell their parents about it when it happened. I was determined not to be like that. When it happened, I would march into my mother's room like the goddamn adult I was, and I would announce it with pride.

'Mother,' I would say, because menstruation meant you were entitled to address your parents in formal salutations, 'I have commenced menstruating!'

In a revelation that will surprise no one, it didn't quite pan out this way. I did go to speak to my mother, but at the last moment I chickened out. It wasn't that I was ashamed. It was that I wanted to keep the secret to myself for a little while longer. I held it to myself tightly, this thing that connected me with a long line of other bleeding bodies, and I revelled in the quiet of it for just a few hours more.

Unfortunately, it turns out I wasn't that good at concealing the secret. I had thought myself an expert on menstruation, in theory at least if not in practice. What I didn't know was that you couldn't flush sanitary pads down the toilet. In common parlance, this is what is known as A Bad Idea. In fact,

FOREWARD

I learned this sometime later that evening, when my mother entered the living room and interrupted a particularly tense scene on *The Bill* and demanded to know if my sister had been responsible for corrupting Norfolk's sewerage system.

'No,' she sneered. She was sixteen and had recently become fluent in the language of snarky teen.

'Clementine?' my mother, asked, turning to me.

'Yes, I whispered in a small voice, my brother and father looking on. 'It was me.'

To say this was mortifying would be an understatement. It wasn't so much that my family knew I had crossed over into adulthood. It was that I had so decidedly cocked up the transition. I didn't know anything about anything!

Still, I consider my experience with menstruation to be overwhelmingly positive which seemingly puts me in a minority camp. According to the data collated by the wonderful folks behind *About Bloody Time*, a majority of young menstruators feel unprepared to deal with their first period and certainly don't experience the same level of joy and belonging that I did. In some circumstances the shame that surrounds menstruation spills out into daily life.

When I was fourteen or fifteen, I remember hearing about a younger girl who had experienced the ultimate humiliation while travelling to school on a bus. She had recently started her period, and her mother had put together a care package of sorts for her. A clean, fresh pair of underwear. A stack of pads. Some painkillers. That kind of thing. It's an act drenched in love and pride. But on the bus that morning, the girl was targeted by bullies. Her bag was snatched and emptied in the aisles, the pads and underwear landing on the floor for everyone to see.

To this day, I'm not sure if this was an urban legend or something that actually happened. But the horror of it is visceral nonetheless. Because every single one of us who bleeds can imagine what it feels like to have someone shame us for that. Many of us have experienced that shame firsthand. We know what it's like to have the sites of our bodies turned into objects of ridicule and disgust. To know that our leaking, seeping, undulating flesh is considered repulsive and unruly. That as long as we experience this expulsion, we are foul, smelly, disgusting – but that once our body ceases to produce these effects, we are also broken somehow.

We know what that feels like.

This is why a work like *About Bloody Time* is so important. The effort, time and skill that Karen Pickering and Jane Bennett have put into collating this essential text cannot be underestimated. To be able to have a conversation as honest as this is so necessary, and to have it curated by the Victorian Women's Trust is a profound gift. I am so proud to be associated with this work, and to collectively work towards a future in which shame and fear are no longer associated with bodily functions as straight-forward as menstruation and menopause.

My period has signified so many things for me throughout my life. Adulthood. Growth. Fertility. It allowed me to have a baby, the child that has become the most important thing to me in my life. I pay homage to it. I will mourn it when it's gone, I'm sure.

These are just my feelings. But maybe they're yours too. I hope so.

Clementine Ford, March 2019

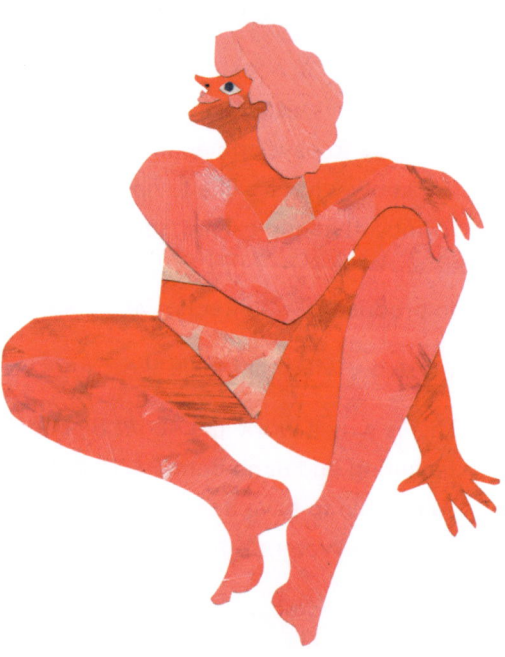

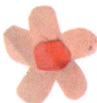

Introduction

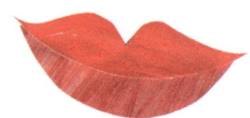

The power of the menstrual cycle is undeniable. Quite literally, our entire existence is guaranteed by it. When women menstruate, they hold within their bodies the power of creation. If nobody menstruated, none of us would be here. It's as simple and as complicated as that.

Menstruation is experienced physically, emotionally and psychologically, but often in ways that are unnecessarily traumatic and difficult for many women. In these pages, we'll share personal experiences, sociocultural analysis and undeniable facts, while we demonstrate that menstruation cuts across the lived experience of women in untold and unexamined ways. We explain how women's lives are punctuated and structured by their menstrual journey, and importantly how the silence and stigma created and maintained by a menstrual taboo harms everyone, but especially girls and women. This menstrual taboo consistently punishes women simply because of their bodies. It is hard to embrace with pride or enthusiasm the idea of bodily autonomy when the cultural messaging is that your bodies are objects of mistrust, dubious hygiene and even loathing. In these ways and more women are conditioned to see their bodies as a liability.

History is full of moments where women saw an opportunity to change the way things were, where they banded together, grabbed that chance and changed the world. A good plan for instigating social change starts with being grounded in the realities of the issue or problem; researching, consulting and communicating broadly with affected groups, from diverse backgrounds and across age groups. Give them a chance to speak and be heard, create a safe space for them and commit to listening and faithfully recording their views and opinions. Ask them how they feel, what they want and how to help. Analyse that data assiduously and look for the patterns of meaning. Find the desire lines through this issue – where do they begin and end? Present these findings in clear and concise ways, not being afraid of the occasional ambivalence and committing fully to the complexity. Gather established and respected experts in the field and work closely with them to maintain the integrity of your analysis. Research the history of your subject, the literature available and contribute meaningfully to the archive. Open the floor. Listen. Hear. Tell the story. Do the work.

INTRODUCTION

This is what we've done. We are going to tell you the story of menstruation and menopause from the perspective of thousands of women, but also situate it within a biological, political, social and cultural context.

We began by extensively researching the topic, building our own exhaustive literature review, about the experience of menstruation and menopause, here in Australia and overseas. We designed a major survey and, in the end, received over 3,000 responses. We asked about first periods, reflections on periods since. We asked about menopause. We asked how women obtained basic information about menstruation and menopause. We asked what would make things easier. We took the same approach throughout a series of 22 discussion groups with women and girls, in this case, across Victoria.

Reading the individual stories gave us a sense of the bigger picture but collating the data and producing statistics proved it categorically: we were shocked and not a little distressed by the clarity of what we found.

Girls and women find menstruation embarrassing and upsetting. So many women and so many girls report in the negative about their menstrual cycle, their experience of menopause, the state of their knowledge and understanding, the treatment accorded to them by others, and their feelings of ignorance, shame, awkwardness and humiliation.

How could it be that one of the most natural things in the world could be understood and experienced as gross and unmentionable? The views across generations were very similar too.

Period prejudice it seems, is deeply ingrained and felt in a contemporary world of such relative sophistication and modernity. But with so many burning issues to capture our attention and occupy our minds, why is this one worthy of our energy and activist impulses, right now?

Firstly, it's long overdue. There has been a paucity of productive, open, honest conversations in the public sphere about menstruation and what it means for women as equals in our society. Many factors contributed to the impossibility of this until now. But the dam has broken. There is no way to justify a continuation of the secrecy, shame and stigma that women live with, as menstruators, in a world that denies their bodies and minimises their power. The harm done to women because of this collective fear and loathing must come to an end.

Second, menstrual silence, shame, ignorance and awkwardness is not only counter to women's fundamental health and wellbeing, but also to the realisation of their full human rights – to be able to avail themselves of the opportunities and resources in life, to live without discrimination; and to be able to participate fully and freely as citizens and consumers in their communities, workplaces and society at large. A world in which women are relegated and demeaned by negative attitudes concerning their bodies can never be an equal world.

ABOUT BLOODY TIME

There is no real and lasting social change without organising and agitating, so by the time you finish reading this book you'll have information and context, and hopefully you'll also have righteous anger to fuel you. It might mean that you commit to changing the culture in your own home, but maybe also your workplace or sporting club. You will have a new way of seeing and talking about menstruation that will inspire courage and clarity in your expressions to others. You'll know that this is one of the great opportunities to close the equality gap between genders and allow women to enjoy the same rights and freedoms as men in our society. You'll be convinced that by developing and implementing a progressive and holistic menstrual awareness education program in schools, workplaces and government, we'll change the future for girls and women, and give boys and men the chance to fully support equality too. We have the slightly immodest but completely achievable goal of guiding the national conversation, revolutionising collective knowledge of women's bodies and bringing about meaningful and lasting social change.

We are living in a time of real impetus and momentum when it comes to women's rights. The right to be free from violence, in our homes, workplaces and all public spaces. The right to equal pay for equal work. The right to have our unpaid labour recognised and valued. The right to empowered and fulfilling sex lives. The right to positive pregnancies, good births and supported motherhood. The right to equal representation and access to power. And the right to live in our bodies without seeing them as incorrect or substandard in any way.

A positive menstrual culture is a key to help us unlock so many of these seemingly intractable issues.

When girls are taught to see their bodies as incredible and powerful, we can break cycles of body hatred and low self-esteem. When women are able to inhabit their bodies with dignity and pride, they can make better choices for themselves, expect more from their relationships, and fully come into their power. Because it's about bloody time.

> *Periods have had some lousy press over the last few thousand years. They've apparently made us unclean, dumb, weak, bad, mad, dangerous or just plain difficult, and have been used as a reason to deny us education and political, economic and spiritual power. Even today, despite relatively good health education most women are still embarrassed about it and, unlike sex, it's still not a topic for comfortable public discussion. For periods to have accrued so much negativity, one thing that you can be assured of is that something very interesting, even powerful, has to be going on.[i]*

Alexandra Pope and Jane Bennett

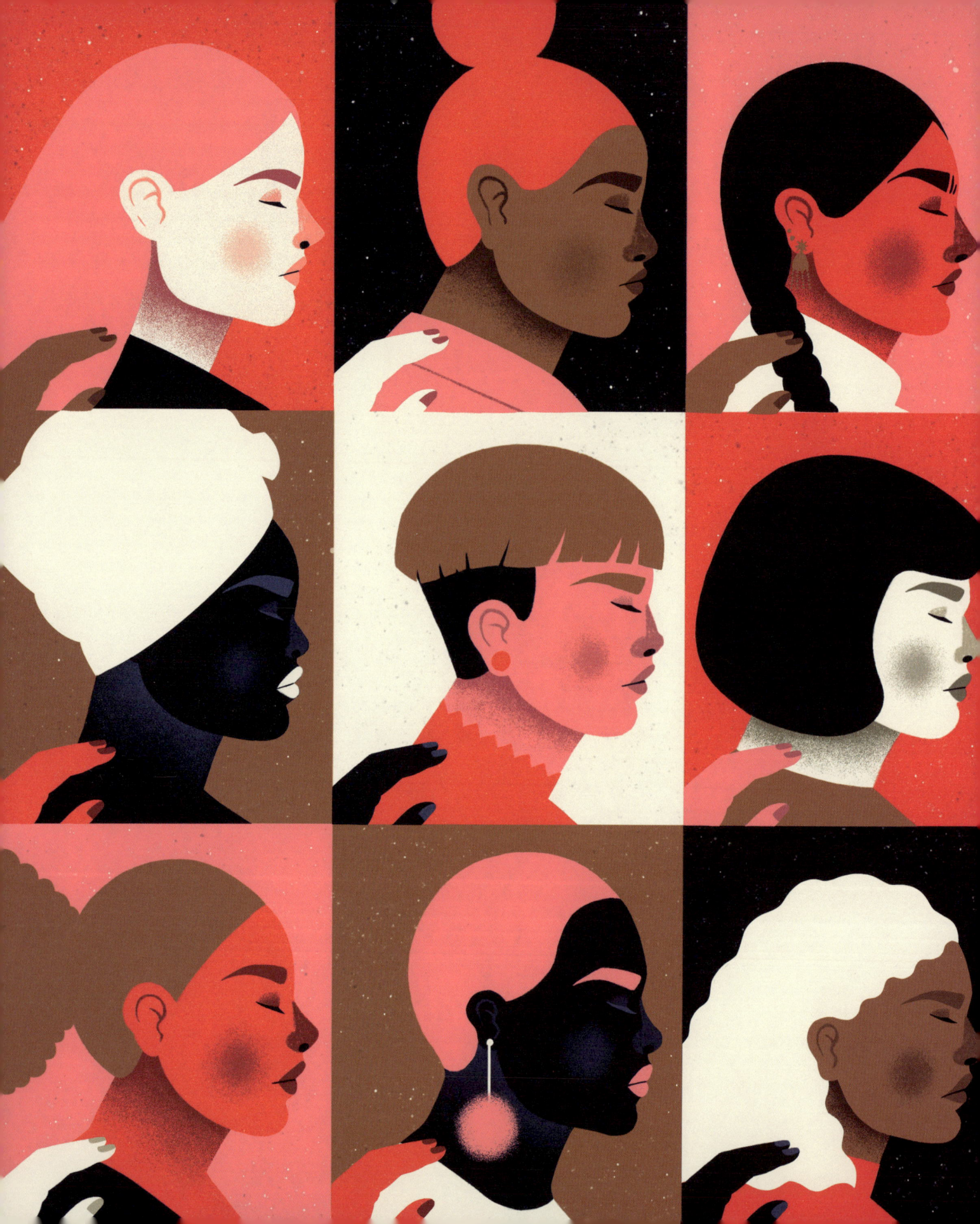

OUR DATA

REACHING OUT TO OVER THREE THOUSAND women and girls about their experience of menstruation and menopause was an ambitious enterprise. We expected it to be revealing and enlightening. We've also been moved and shocked.

What we have now is an important and unique body of data. Our findings are significant because of the size of the study, and the broad scope that included girls and women of diverse ages and backgrounds, from around the world. But also, crucially, it was designed to invite women and girls to speak openly, in spaces that were supportive and safe, and help them reflect on their experience in a way many never had before. We wanted to know how girls and women felt about their menstrual cycle, what they thought of it, and in valuing women's own reflections and experiences, this separates our data from much of what we discovered in our literature review, clinical trials and academic research. A major difference is that part of our process enabled women and girls to listen and be heard, as well as connect with one another and feel validated.

We conducted an online questionnaire survey and facilitated face-to-face discussion groups for girls and women across key demographics and locations. The questionnaire survey included multiple choice and invitations to provide open-ended commentary, which allowed for self-guided reflection and for observations that didn't necessarily fit neatly into a question-and-answer format.

Approximately three and a half thousand girls and women took part in our survey. These were broken into four age groups – girls aged 12-18 years, teenagers and women aged 19-30 years, women aged 31-45 and women aged 46+. The majority of questionnaire respondents came from Australia and New Zealand, followed by Canada, the USA and the UK, with a small number of respondents from a further 51 countries.

3460 women and girls were surveyed:

- 🔴 12-18 years 6.5%
- 🔴 19-30 years 22.7%
- 🔴 31-45 years 34.9%
- ⚫ 46 & over 35.9%

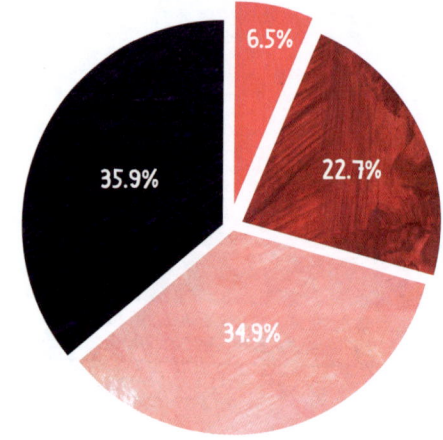

OUR DATA

They came from:

- ● Australia & New Zealand 60.8%
- ● Canada & the USA 30.1%
- ● United Kingdom 3.8%
- ● 51 other countries. 5.3%

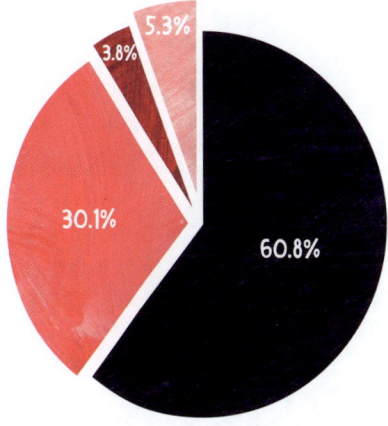

We also conducted twenty-two discussion groups across Victoria mirroring the survey age groupings. These discussions were generally over two hours and deliberately included suburban and regional settings. All sessions were recorded and transcribed while guaranteeing anonymity.

We realise this sampling of women is technically not random and cannot be considered wholly representative. Nonetheless we are confident of the power of so many women's accounts. There is a point at which patterns in responses within such a mass can be relied upon to start important conversations and prompt further exploration.

Overall, we ended up with an extraordinarily rich yield of both qualitative and quantitative material, painstakingly processed and distilled.

This mix of qualitative and quantitative data shows that across generations of menstruating and menopausal women, the story is relatively bleak. For most girls and women, their experience is not pleasant, joyous or positive.

The experience of menstruation is often marred by negativity, which then carries on throughout so many women's lives and which insidiously affects their sense of self, their confidence, awareness of their physical bodies and emotional realms, their sexual decision-making, and the management of their relationships at home and in workplaces.

The quantitative picture: some hard facts

We asked girls and women how they felt generally about their periods. Seven in ten girls aged 12-18 years had negative feelings about their periods – four out of ten disliked everything about their periods, three in ten saw their periods as good and bad but were still 'mostly bad'.

> "As a teenager I **suffered in silence** for too long with period pain. I still went to school when I had it but wasn't really listening or learning anything because **I was so distracted.** I was too shy to discuss it with my mum or GP."

OUR DATA

As a teenager I suffered in silence for too long with period pain. I still went to school when I had it but wasn't really listening or learning anything because I was so distracted I was too shy to discuss it with my mum or GP (General Practitioner).

At school it was awful to have a heavy period. I remember getting blood on my school dress and sitting in the bathroom for hours painting whiteout over the stains. High school is a scary and judgemental place if something goes wrong.

It took me many years to be relaxed about periods. I felt very ashamed of bleeding as a teenager.

Even going to an all girls' school, the notion that someone had their period was made out by other girls to be disgusting. Although every girl in the year obviously had to go through the same thing, it would be absolutely horrifying to have to ask your friend if you could borrow a tampon or pad. It made me feel embarrassed about having it and obsessed about maintaining secrecy.

Across all age groups over forty per cent expressed predominantly negative sentiments, including seventeen per cent disliking everything about it. Twenty-two per cent were ambivalent as to whether periods are good or bad. One in four felt predominantly positive, while a little over one in ten liked everything about it.

How did they feel about their period?

All ages

- ● Dislike everything.........................17%
- ● Some good and bad but mostly bad........25%
- ● Neither predominately good nor bad......22%
- ● Some good and bad but mostly good.......25%
- ● Like everything..........................11%

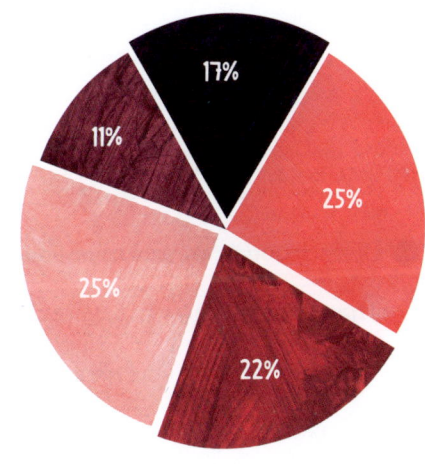

Girls aged 12 to 18:

- Dislike everything. 41%
- Some good and bad but mostly bad. 29%
- Neither predominantly good or bad. 20%
- Some good and bad but mostly good. 8%
- Like everything. 2%

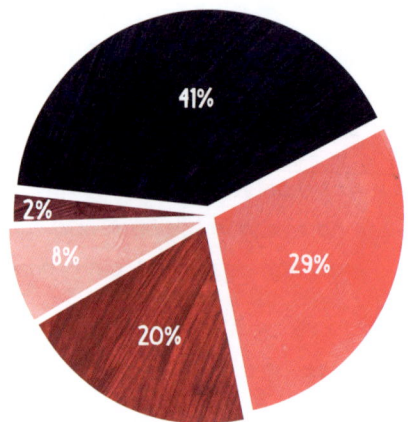

We asked where they were when the first bleeding started and what they thought might be happening. The majority of our respondents were at home when their first period started, while sixteen percent were at school and the rest elsewhere. Two thirds said yes, they understood what was happening, a quarter thought they knew but were a bit uncertain and nearly one in ten had no idea.

Where were they when their period first started:

- Home. 65%
- School. 16%
- Elsewhere. 19%

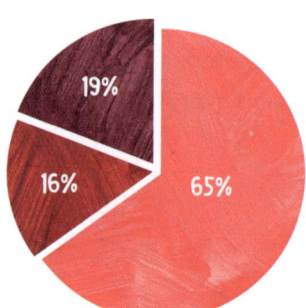

Did they know what was happening:

- Understood what was happening. 66%
- Thought they knew but were a bit uncertain. 25%
- Had no idea what was happening. 9%

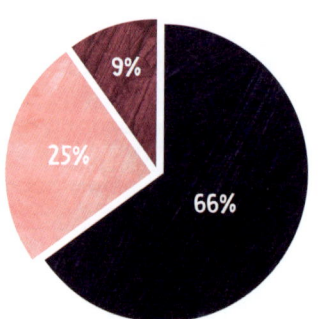

We asked whether they felt prepared for their first period. Over half felt they were not, around a third indicated they were 'somewhat prepared' and more than one in ten felt they were as prepared as they needed to be.

We were keen to establish respondent's sources of menstrual information. In the main, while they were able to nominate multiple sources, the primary sources across age groups were mothers (more than three in four), followed by school (well over fifty per cent, with significant jumps in percentages for each age group – forty-four per cent of women 46 and over to sixty-seven percent of girls 12 to 18 sourced information from school). Next came friends at nearly four in ten, and books, nearly three in ten. Not surprisingly, girls aged 12 to 18 years nominated the internet more than other groups with fifteen per cent using this resource, but this was still minor compared with mothers, schools and friends.

All age groups received information about menstruation from these sources:

- Mother 77%
- School 56%
- Friends 38%
- Books 22%

We also wanted to establish how women felt about menopause; their preparedness, sources of information, and what would have improved their experience. More than one in four felt happy about reaching menopause, a little over a third acknowledged some negative aspects but were happy overall about doing so, thirteen percent were reasonably neutral, feeling that it was neither good nor bad, while nearly a quarter expressed dislike of everything about it. One in four women felt prepared, while nearly three in ten felt only somewhat prepared. Close to a half felt they were unprepared. Far and away the most important source of information were friends for over half; followed by doctors, the internet and television each a little over four in ten women. Books were useful for one in five women and magazines for fewer than that. Seventeen per cent of women found their mother's support helpful, and seven per cent their sisters.

How did they feel about having reached menopause?

- Happy about it 27%
- Positive and negative but overall happy 36%
- Neither negative nor positive 13%
- Positive and negative but overall unenjoyable. 1%
- Dislike everything about it 23%

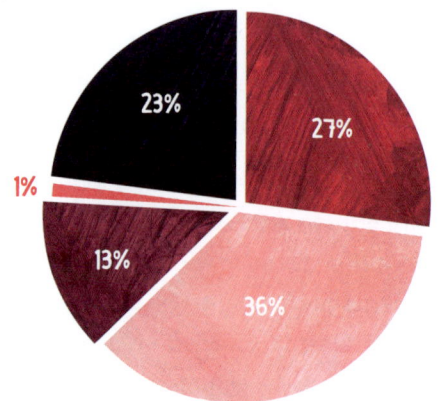

Did they feel that they were prepared for menopause?

- Felt prepared 25%
- Somewhat prepared 28.5%
- Felt unprepared 46.5%

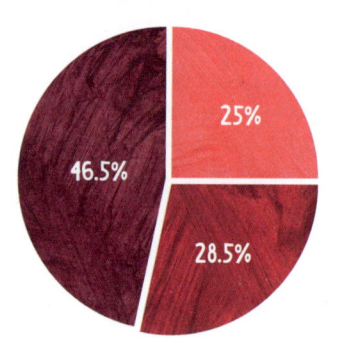

Sources of information about menopause:

- Friends 51%
- Doctors 42%
- Internet 42%
- Television 41%
- Books 20%
- Mother 17%
- Magazines 16%
- Sister 7%

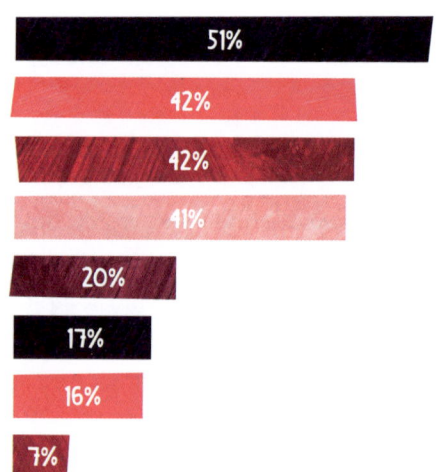

OUR DATA

In terms of what would have improved their experience of menopause, more than one in three women nominated reliable information, followed by one in four choosing being able to take time off. A similar number would have liked being able to talk openly about it and over one in five nominated not having to make excuses for feeling hot or tired and close to one in five chose being able to ask for what was needed from either a partner or employer.

What would make the transition to menopause a better experience?

- Reliable information 36%
- Ability to take time off when needed 26%
- Being able to speak openly 25%
- Not needing to make excuses 21%
- Being able to ask for help 18%

Finally, we sought views on what would make menstruation a better experience. We listed multiple choices, which ranged from a day off to rest, cheaper pads and tampons, talking openly about periods, not having to make excuses when feeling unwell, being able to ask for what was needed and not feeling shame when buying sanitary products. Generally, for all age groups, close to six in ten nominated time to rest, and nearly four in ten would appreciate cheaper menstrual products. Thirty per cent of women wanted to be able to talk more openly about periods, more than a third wanted to no longer make excuses when they felt unwell while menstruating, nearly a quarter would like to be able to ask for what they needed from a partner or employer, and almost one in four wanted to be able to buy menstrual products without feeling shame.

What would make their period a better experience?

- ● Time to rest 58%
- ● Cheaper menstrual products 37%
- ● Not need to make excuses 35%
- ● Be able to talk more openly 30%
- ● Be able to ask for what I need from a partner or employer 24%
- ● Be able to buy menstrual products without shame 23%

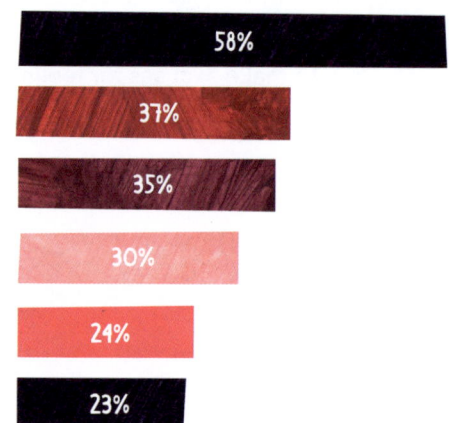

A qualitative picture: a rich vein of commentary

Facts and figures are important. But we also know that there is nothing like discussion and close listening to deepen our awareness and understanding of the matters at hand.

We not only listened closely to several hundred girls and women in group sessions around Victoria, but we also provided opportunities throughout the survey questionnaire for them to comment freely and in detail. We were amply rewarded.

First period pain

From these discussion groups and questionnaire comments, most women and girls commented that getting their first period made them variously feel shocked, scared, embarrassed, worried, awkward, disgusted, terrified, panicked, angry, secretive and ashamed. Did they know what was happening? Not necessarily. Was it their period or something else? Not totally sure. Where did they find menstrual products and how were they to use them? What of the colour, consistency and quantity of menstrual blood? How long did a period last? How often would all this occur? All these questions led to guesswork as girls were afraid of telling others, anxious about people 'knowing', and nonplussed about what their body was doing and what this all meant. Many were confused by the sight of blood. Some recalled great loneliness if they were the first of their group to get their period, or if they didn't know whether others were yet menstruating.

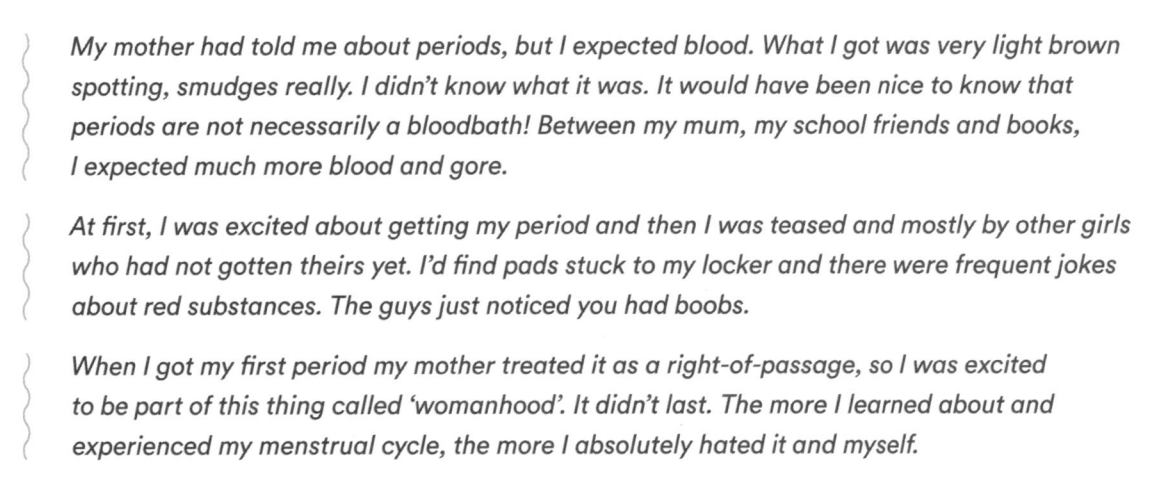

> *My mother had told me about periods, but I expected blood. What I got was very light brown spotting, smudges really. I didn't know what it was. It would have been nice to know that periods are not necessarily a bloodbath! Between my mum, my school friends and books, I expected much more blood and gore.*

> *At first, I was excited about getting my period and then I was teased and mostly by other girls who had not gotten theirs yet. I'd find pads stuck to my locker and there were frequent jokes about red substances. The guys just noticed you had boobs.*

> *When I got my first period my mother treated it as a right-of-passage, so I was excited to be part of this thing called 'womanhood'. It didn't last. The more I learned about and experienced my menstrual cycle, the more I absolutely hated it and myself.*

Some described feeling annoyed, trapped, burdened and sad about new restrictions. Cramps, heavy bleeding, extreme tiredness and nausea were new sensations, along with feeling moody and emotional. On a more positive note, others expressed relief that their period had arrived (finally!); that they were 'normal', 'grown up' and 'could have kids'.

> *One day when I was thirteen I was called to the nurse's office at school because my mother had discovered brown spots in my underwear while she was doing the laundry. The nurse told me that I was 'spotting' and I had no idea what she was talking about. She gave me a pad, but I didn't know what I was supposed to do with it. I felt so confused and stupid and still feel badly for my girl self. Even now one of my deepest insecurities is 'not being intelligent', which stems from the humiliation I felt at not having noticed or recognised my first period when it came.*

Some felt it was no big deal. Some celebrated alone or with their families and judged things as natural and normal. With a few years distance, girls tended to remember the experience of their first period somewhat more positively. Many women reflected on the difficulty of their own experience, remembering the products they were presented with, like torn up old sheets, a used sanitary belt and plastic pants, or massive pads, and they vowed to do things very differently for their own daughters.

> *When I was eleven, I went to a special day about periods and puberty with my mum. Although I was embarrassed at first it turned out to be really fun, and I think it was enlightening for my mum too. Afterwards I felt really close to her and we had so many amazing conversations about periods, from stories about her experiences to finding out information about products and how things work. We laughed a lot. It was like we'd joined a special club together. This certainly helped me navigate the sometimes difficult experiences of the next few years.*

Periods since: more of the same

Mostly, irrespective of age, women expressed dislike and negativity. They described physical and emotional pain and difficulty that accompanied their periods – plenty to alert institutions and professionals involved with health and wellbeing to the impact periods have on women.

> *As a teenager I used to vomit my cramps were so bad. At school I'd just run out of the classroom, throw up, and come back to finish the day. It was horrible, but I never considered I could go home from school, nor did anyone suggest it. We were made to feel that it's something to hide, yet something to be happy about, yet something to pretend isn't happening, yet something to celebrate our womanhood. It was very confusing.*
>
> *Even though we were told periods were a natural part of being a woman, the other message was just suck it up and carry on. Intellectually I know better, but I still push myself when I feel exhausted or crampy and would benefit greatly from slowing down or having an early night. It's like I have a voice in my head that judges me for being weak and indulgent. I'm slowly unwinding this legacy, but it's a battle every month.*

Women described their struggle with the pressures of work and family and the ways that difficult premenstrual or menstrual symptoms added to their overall stress and tiredness. Many women

"
Even though we were told periods were a natural part of being a woman, the other message was just **suck it up and carry on.** Intellectually I know better, but I still push myself when I feel exhausted or crampy and would benefit greatly from slowing down or having an early night. It's like I have a voice in my head that judges me for being weak and indulgent. **I'm slowly unwinding this legacy,** but it's a battle every month.
"

who suffer from Polycystic ovarian syndrome (PCOS), endometriosis and fibroids indicated they were tired of the debilitating and life-diminishing experience and are frustrated by the lack of improvement. Others have embraced supportive lifestyle practices and/or specific therapies, which seemed to transform their periods and enhance their general well-being. Compared with younger women, many older women seemed also to have discovered the value of rest and self-care, as well as asking for support or time off during their period. While still experiencing their menstrual cycle, some women expressed excitement about their forthcoming menopause as heralding a new stage of life, whereas others were anxious about menopausal symptoms and distressed that menopause suggests they were getting old.

> *For years I hated and was confused by my period, my reproductive system and my body generally. In my early twenties I was having regular sex with my boyfriend and, being terrified of getting pregnant, was on the Pill. In my thirties I was diagnosed with Polycystic ovarian syndrome and struggled with my weight and my body image and was chronically anxious. I was also struggling to get pregnant. When I began fertility treatment I had a beautiful realisation – I was supposed to love and cherish my body and its amazing reproductive processes! I began acupuncture, limited dairy and sugar, increased organic and healthful eating, and started exercising regularly. I was able to conceive naturally and adored my pregnancy. Now I see great value in loving my body and honouring all of its beautiful abilities.*

Family background

Not surprisingly, mums, dads and families were seen as significantly impacting on women's experience of periods, and, to a lesser degree, of menopause. But again, it was more negative than positive. A lot described their experience in bleak terms of 'taboo', of feeling awkward, ashamed and embarrassed. Many said they lacked connection, support and information; and that their family culture contributed to their negative experience of menstruation.

> *I was taught to hide it and never show weakness.*

> *In my family periods were never talked about. So, I never talked about it, and still don't if I can possibly help it. Over the last couple of years, I developed excessive bleeding from*

> *fibroids and recently went to a gynaecologist for the first time. It was extremely humiliating and distressing for me. I feel overwhelmed now just thinking about it.*

Quite a number of women in their 40s reflected on their youth and saw more clearly now how repressive religious, traditional or male-dominated family situations caused them to feel alone, ashamed, ostracised, sad, uninformed, unprepared, embarrassed, and weaker and less valuable than boys and men. In a related vein, some women wrote about fathers and brothers who judged and teased. Many women described having worked to overcome the negative conditioning they received about their body from their family, culture and religion.

> *My family is very comfortable talking about periods, contraception, conceiving and menopause, which means sometimes I am overly comfortable talking about it to other people.*

> *Nothing was ever explicit, but somehow, I picked up from a very young age that the male gender was superior and the female weak.*

> *I come from a long line of pretty savvy women and I went to a girls' school, so all things period have always been a pretty normal, shame-free part of my life. I fondly remember the care and attention I received from my mum when I got my period.*

A strong theme in the qualitative commentary revolved around the pressure faced by women to 'soldier on' or 'just get on with it'. Periods were no reason to shirk responsibilities, even in the face of difficult menstrual symptoms like pain, exhaustion or heavy bleeding.

In families where there was greater openness and support, fathers, brothers and boyfriends were helpful as well as the girl's mothers and sisters. They learnt that menstruation and menopause were natural, normal and healthy, positive aspects of womanhood. In other instances, though, women described their irritation at having been demeaned and shamed by partners, teased and goaded with comments about periods, PMS (Pre-Menstrual Syndrome), mood swings and being 'hormonal'. Some women watched their mothers suffer a difficult menopause, and for some, hysterectomy had been so common in their families that they had no familial examples of non-surgical menopause to guide them.

The prospect of menopause

Turning to menopause, women related a wide range of feelings. For many, both extremes featured at once: sad and excited, happy and anxious, worried and 'can't wait'.

Many women were concerned about aging skin, loss of libido and attractiveness, hot flushes and sleeplessness, mood changes, weight and changing body shape. Another concern, loss of fertility, was an issue of identity for some, and a loss of potential for others.

Some women were put off and frightened by what they read while others commented that reading and attending workshops helped them prepare for and positively frame menopause. Others found it difficult to find the information they wanted, and many were concerned about how they would manage as they begin to experience the symptoms of peri-menopause.

> *I did not really understand the extent to which menopause would affect my sex life. When I spoke to a male doctor about my lack of sex drive he said, 'Oh well, you have had all your children now so it shouldn't be an issue'!*

> *At first, I mourned the changes in my body: hot flashes happened at the most inconvenient times, night sweats were a major problem. Then one day I made up my mind to stay as busy as possible so that I wouldn't be depressed. I built a terraced stonewall in my driveway in six months, which I call The Great Wall of Menopause! Keep busy is the best advice I can give.*

Many found the physical and emotional changes associated with menopause trying, especially the loss of libido and a dry, thin-walled vagina, ongoing hot flushes, fuzzy-headedness and loss of coherent thought, poor sleep, irritability, being on an emotional roller-coaster and general exhaustion. Some expressed grief at the loss of fertility and the possibility of babies and said that they missed their periods.

Other women shared the relief and joy they felt about no longer having periods or having to worry about pregnancy, the absence of period pain and no more inconvenient heavy bleeding. Many described feeling liberated, more in control and more alive, and overall expressed positivity about the transformative and empowering shift to a new stage of life that menopause represented.

While a number of women were glad for their supportive friends and family, others were sorry that there was so little positive and helpful information and treatment available and that in their experience menopause was rarely talked about. Postmenopausal women identified the need for greater understanding, support, open communication, acceptance, normalisation and respect.

What would make things easier?

Overall, our open-ended commentary boxes were filled with further evidence of the way women felt spectacularly disadvantaged by the combination of their cyclic life and work; a fact that in all likelihood diminished their overall productivity, creativity and agency at work, not to mention pleasure and comfort in the work environment.

While time to rest and greater openness and support were popular recommendations, a number of women described choosing to work on a self-employed basis because of the difficulties of managing their menstrual needs in previous workplaces. Many others shared experiences of being the butt of jokes or derision, for example, being 'on the rag', 'hormonal' or 'menopausal', and not feeling able to be honest if they needed support or time off for difficult symptoms.

> *Sometimes I'm really unwell with my period but feel I can't be honest about it because they'll think I'm 'weak' or 'being a princess' for not being able to cope. When it's so bad that I need to take a day off work I lie about why.*

> *On the first day of my period I often have a migraine and terrible cramping, which certainly makes for a rough workday. It would be nice to be able to call in 'sick' if I needed to without fear of backlash.*

Girls commented about wanting an end to periods being used to tease or bully them. They also described how they would prefer not to be anxious about leaking and being obvious about having a period. They wrote of being worried whether they could find a bin or have easy access to pads or tampons when they needed them.

> *I still feel like I have to sneak my used pads and tampons to the bin because there is some kind of grossness about it.*

> *I always feel embarrassed when I have to heavily wrap and dispose of my tampon in someone else's kitchen bin.*

> *The worst experiences were when I got my period and didn't have any tampons or pads with me. I felt stressed, embarrassed to ask for help and worried that other people could see stains.*

Older woman identified a number of things which would have helped them when they were younger. These included better information and practical and emotional support, especially the latter. They wanted an end to menstrual shame. They wanted boys and men to be more informed and understanding. They wanted to see doctors trained in, and with more understanding of, menopause, and more able to offer alternatives to drugs or surgery.

Better health treatment would help

Many women nominated the attitudes of health professionals they'd seen as adding significantly to their suffering. They felt dismissed, pressured, ashamed and frustrated. Women spoke about their experiences of PMS, Premenstrual Dysmorphic Disorder (PMDD) and the intensification of emotions and existing mental health problems before or during their period, especially in terms of what did and didn't help. Severity of pain and heavy bleeding was such for a number of women that these symptoms impacted their mental health.

Feeling heard and empathetically understood was often missing, as was useful information and options. In other cases, women found relief and regained 'their life' after years of suffering when they found a helpful practitioner, diagnosis and treatment. At times, women found relief from symptoms through a wide range of treatments and self-care practices, sometimes taking a considerable time to find what worked for them. For some a healthy diet, nutritional supplements, herbs, yoga, gym and other exercise, counselling, naturopathy, Chinese medicine, changing their attitude toward their body and processes, and learning menstrual cycle awareness all helped. While for other women it was finding relief using the Pill, an IUD (intrauterine device) or HRT (hormone replacement therapy).

> *I was violently ill and had severe cramping, extreme migraines, diarrhoea, vomiting, was nauseous, angry, depressed, crying, moody, cranky, unable to walk, with horrible back*

and abdominal pain, severe and heavy bleeding, dizzy and fainting, craving chocolate and hot tea as well as red meat, and had swollen ankles and weak knees. I bled for ten to fourteen days each month and had massive blood clots. There were times I felt like someone wearing steel-toed boots was kicking me in my back. I would rock back and forth crying and was unable to converse properly or think rationally. I was exhausted and unable to function. Several times I passed out at Junior High and had to be rushed to hospital by ambulance. Then just before my thirteenth birthday I was put on birth control pills to control the excessive bleeding. It didn't fix everything but certainly helped me to have a more normal life.

Disability and menstruation

We asked women 'If you identify as having a disability what impact has this had on your experience of periods and menopause?'. We make no claim that the answers women gave are in any way broadly representative, due to the sample being small and the diversity of their disabling conditions. That said, women's responses were nonetheless enlightening and instructive, a place from which further enquiry and greater menstrual and menopausal support could begin.

While most women who identify as having a disability did not see this as having an impact on their periods, most commonly this was because the disability manifested late in their menstrual career. For other women having a period was made more difficult because of their impaired mobility, cyclic hormones causing chronic inflammation to spike, visual impairment making it hard to see and manage menstrual blood, body awareness and mental health issues exacerbating paranoia about menstrual hygiene, and difficulty in learning how to manage periods.

For some women their mental health condition, particularly anxiety and depression, is significantly affected by their menstrual cycle, both pre-menstrually and menstrually. One woman said, 'periods definitely make my depression worse' and a woman with low vision commented, 'when I have my period I don't know whether I am dripping blood around bathrooms or if I've been able to clean my clothes and sheets well enough'. For another menopausal symptoms multiplied many times the difficulty she experienced in managing her disability. For her poor understanding and inadequate treatment options from health professionals made an unpleasant situation much worse.

Where does this lead us?

It was our privilege to receive the trust of the thousands of girls and women who responded to the survey and participated in the discussion groups. As such, we have taken great care to present both the quantitative and qualitative data in a way that is both rigorous and genuinely reflects the diverse responses and stories we received.

The findings are clear. Women and girls describe an experience of menarche (the first period) and menstruation often shot through with a kind of collective anxiety. Despite the best efforts of individuals (both private and professional), menarche, menstruation and menopause still tend to be difficult and traumatic for many girls and women and carry a great deal of negative association.

For many, it means continuing secrecy, anxiety and pain. It can result in alienation from their bodies or from other people, and an atmosphere of shame, reproach and fear. There is a culture of silence around menstruation, and a lack of openness and comfort on the part of adults, contributing to many girls feeling unprepared for their first period. Of the women who were facing or had already experienced menopause, the numbers broke in similar ways. The stigma attached to menstruation in general led to many respondents feeling unprepared for menopause. Not only do women and girls feel negatively about their menstrual cycle but they feel that others do too. The findings also suggest that many women and girls operate from a position of ignorance and disconnection from their bodies. Clearly, we have a massive problem with our collective menstrual culture, and how women and girls experience their menstrual and menopausal lives.

We need to examine this closely.

What produces and sustains such negative emotions in girls and women with regard to their menstrual cycle?

What is at the source of such negativity when the cycle itself, in purely biological terms, contains nothing of the sort?

Menstruation simply is. It is a routine function of certain bodies, and it has a purpose and meaning of its own, despite the cultural narratives surrounding it. Like sneezing, or crying, it's the body's way of getting something done, of moving from one state to another, only in the case of menstruation it is repetitive and predictable (to a degree), thus forming a cycle. The body is inherently cyclical. Every system within it operates by sequence, and most of these are considered neutral. Breath goes in and out, blood moves around and through the body, skin regenerates. The body is staying alive through the endocrine system, which produces the hormones we need for many physical functions, including the ability to reproduce and fulfil the basic evolutionary purpose of all species: survival.

This is how simply our menstrual cycle can be explained and understood, but cultural attitudes around menstruation and menopause are anything but straightforward.

We know that there is a serious vacuum in women's own knowledge about menarche, menstruation and menopause, and that this results in confusion, disconnection and fear for women and girls. We know that a deep chasm exists between the biological facts of menstruation and society's attitude toward it. And we know that there is cognitive dissonance for women and girls who are encouraged to be obsessed with their physical appearance and sexual appeal, while at the same time having little idea what is going on inside their bodies. We have an epidemic of shame surrounding menstruation and menopause, and it's not the fault of individuals. It is historical, structural and cultural.

We need to address two related and equally important issues.

Firstly, women and girls need to know what is happening inside their bodies. In terms of menstruation, this means understanding their sexual and reproductive systems, how they work and why. The choices that women need to make about their bodies are endless, around sex and sexuality, contraception and conception, pregnancy and childbirth, fitness and wellness, diet and exercise, illness and disease, and simply how they live inside their own body. How can they make the right decisions, for themselves and their best interests, if they aren't fully informed? What kind of decisions do you make when you don't have all the facts?

And secondly, we'll look at the menstrual taboo and the proliferation of shame around menstruation, how many myths surround it and why these cultural attitudes are so pervasive and persistent.

In the next section we'll take a deep dive into the physiology of menstruation, to lay out the details, clarify the process, debunk the myths, and provide what our data suggests may be the first comprehensive, plain-language explanation of menstruation and menopause many of our readers have encountered. Put simply, we have created what our respondents dreamed of having access to from a young age, as they told us in the survey – a simple, neutral summary of this relatively straightforward, though no less amazing, process. So many participants expressed their regret and resentment that they were given so little preparation for the different stages of their menstrual lives. We can't go back in time to rectify this, but we can make sure a comprehensive and authoritative explainer exists now. This kind of positive menstrual education can set girls on a path of lifelong learning about their bodies, where their natural curiosity and interest is met with information, encouragement and support. Women who have been taught to check in with their bodies and listen to them can keep developing these skills over a lifetime, with profound impacts on their sense of self-worth, their health and their decision-making.

Then we need to reckon with the menstrual taboo. It's our aim to disrupt its power and dismantle it for good. This requires locating it within different cultures and moments throughout history, but also looking around us now at all the ways it currently manifests in women and girls' lives. The burden of stigma should not be borne any longer. If we can see the menstrual taboo for what it is: a set of cultural attitudes that attaches negativity and shame to menstruation, then we can deconstruct it. This puts us on the path to creating the kind of change that would render it not only less powerful, but also a relic of history.

These two stories are, of course, part of the same larger whole. As long as women are confused about what is going on inside their bodies, they will be susceptible to narratives that attach blame and shame to their physical form. When women and girls have deep and ongoing awareness of how their bodies work, they will value themselves differently, relate to themselves and others differently, and construct their lives differently. They will also have the best inoculation going against the menstrual taboo.

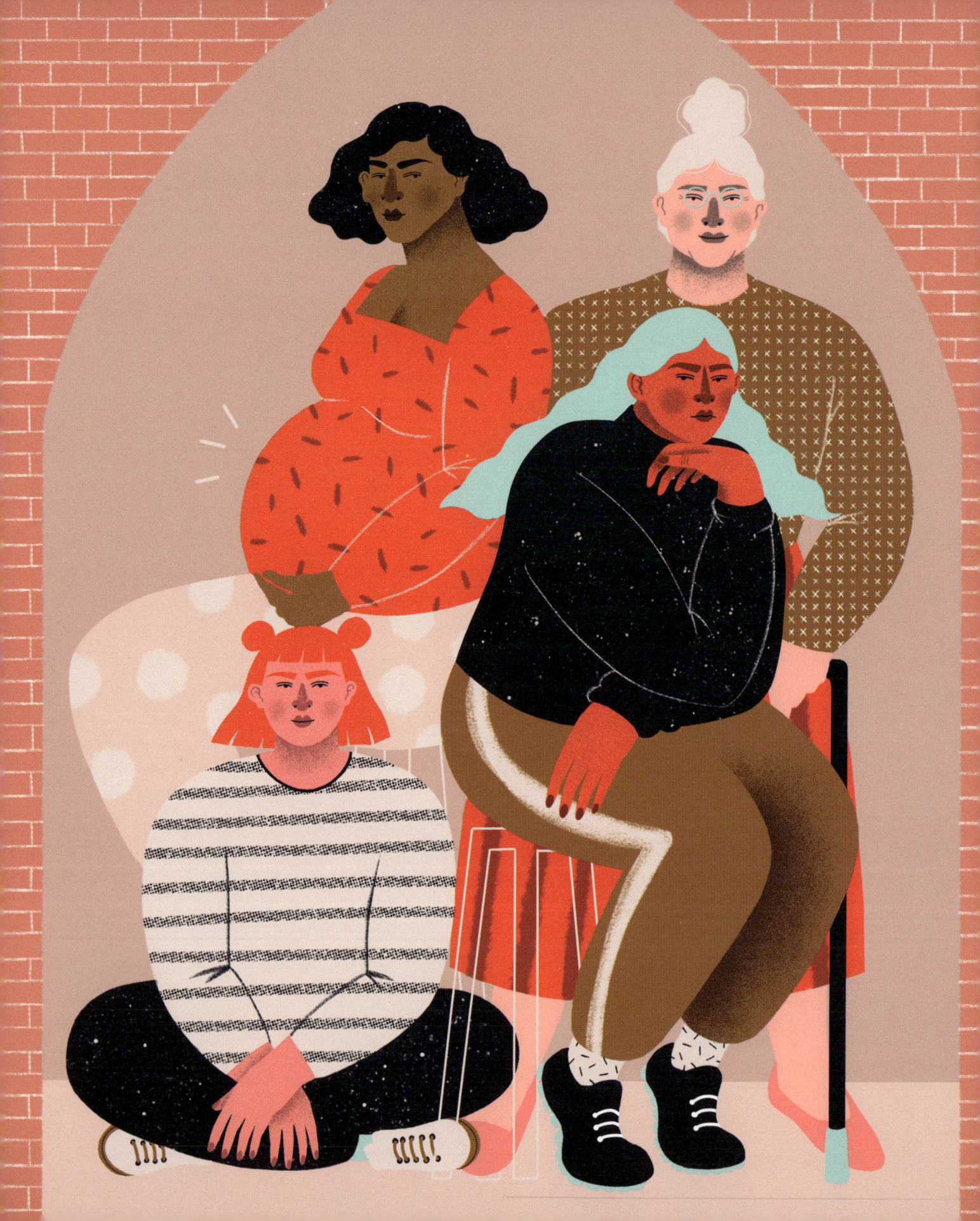

THE BIOLOGICAL INTEGRITY OF MENSTRUATION

WE START OUR SERIOUS EXPLORATION with menstruation and menopause within a biological context – free of other factors at work, such as culture and gender.

In establishing this *biological* context, we want to provide a detailed neutral description of the menstrual cycle that demystifies the complexity, but in ways where readers can feel confident, and increasingly knowledgeable – some for the first time in their lives.

Fertility is fundamental to life, plainly, obviously and indisputably.

We live, we eat, and by virtue of the fertility of plants and animals, we are clothed and to a large extent sheltered by the products of fertility. And, here we are, getting on with our lives, because every one of *our* ancestors was reproductively successful. In this sense ancestry is much more wondrous than a genealogical chart alone can convey.

Every one of our foremothers grew one of our direct ancestors, or in the most recent case *each one of us*, in their womb, and all or almost all birthed vaginally. Some died in the process, many didn't. Whatever the drama, joy or struggle of each of their individual stories *we are here as testimony to this profound ongoing process*. This is not to say we are, or should be, reduced to our reproductive capacity, far from it, however in a discussion of menstruation and fertility we do need to recognise their centrality to our existence, and therefore our collective capacity to do other important things.

Intrinsic to our foremothers' fertility, and therefore to our own life, is their menstrual cycle. Whether they had many children or just one, one thing is certain, their bodies cycled. Signalled by a regular bleed over many years it is by virtue of this cycle, by their periodic bleeding, that we are here. This is a great multitude of mothers and a great ocean of menstruation.

We generally understand menstruation and the menstrual cycle in terms of reproduction; conception, pregnancy and birth. Important stuff certainly. However, as *99.5% of our ovulations will end in menstruation* (for the average woman in a developed country, except where long-term use of hormonal contraception eliminates ovulation) it is surely time for us to think more about menstruation as an important event in and of itself, worthy of our curiosity and respect, study and understanding.

From the get-go

Our own journey of fertility begins well before birth. Early in our development there is no physical or hormonal difference between male and female embryos, other than our microscopic XY and XX chromosomes. At around six to eight weeks in utero gonads, which soon become either ovaries or testicles, are detectable. By seven weeks, the embryo has a 'genital tubercle', 'urogenital groove', and 'labioscrotal folds'. These are the early, unisex internal and external reproductive organs, though the start of customisation is just days away.

During the following five weeks, the foetus begins to produce hormones that cause their proto-sex organs to morph and grow into those that are recognisably male or female. And, for a small but statistically significant number, several conditions can lead to various kinds of intersex development in a foetus. This occurrence is often said to be of a similar percentage to babies born with red hair, that is, between one and two per cent.[i]

However, in most cases the unisex organs are gradually remodelled into ovaries, uterus, vagina, clitoris, and labia in girls, and penis, scrotum, testes, epididymis, vas deferens, and seminal vesicles in boys. By five months in-utero a baby girl has all the (immature) eggs she will ever have, all five to seven *million* of them.[ii] The abundant and intelligently selective nature of fertility being what it is, by birth this number will have reduced to between one and two million. By the time a girl has her first period this will have reduced to around 350,000 eggs.

The fascinating prequel to this biological fact is that the gamete, or immature egg cell, that in part became you, was already inside your birth mother while she was nestled, as yet unborn, inside your grandmother. Ponder that.

> *I'd known about the 'egg that in part became me was inside my mum while she was inside my grandmother' thing for many years, then, one day, when this popped into my mind I rather belatedly made the link with my own family, rather than just as a fact of biology. My maternal grandmother died as a young woman, so I never met her. We only have a few scratchy photos and some sweet stories to know her by. Nonetheless, the egg that, in part, became me had started life nestled deep inside her womb, in one of my own mother's budding ovaries). Suddenly I felt a powerful connection and intimacy with my grandmother, Gladys Irene, which has stayed with me ever since. I think of her often.*

At birth, babies are often still awash with their mother's adult, pregnant, and birthing hormones. As a result, boys may have swollen, erect penises, and a girl's labia may be swollen too, with some having a tiny bleed that looks like a period. Both boys and girls may have swollen nipple buds and lactate. When this happens the milk droplets produced are rather fantastically named 'witch's milk' – another cultural clue that references deep anxieties about female reproductive power. This naturally ebbs in the first weeks of life ex-utero as the important business of babyhood gets underway.

Growing up: puberty

From a biological point of view the major differences between children and adults are a) physical size and b) reproductive maturity, and of course, much else about brains, bones and hormones.

So, for a myriad of reasons, some known and many yet to be discovered, puberty begins. First come surges and cascades of sex hormones, triggered by a small gland in the brain called the hypothalamus, which starts the process by secreting gonadotropinreleasing hormone (GnRH). This in turn stimulates the pituitary gland, a pea-sized organ attached underneath the hypothalamus, which produces two hormones: luteinising hormone (LH) and follicle stimulating hormone (FSH). Once released LH and FSH signal the ovaries to begin releasing oestrogens. There are in fact twelve oestrogens, led by oestradiol, and these initiate the perceivable transformations of puberty in girls.

Luckily for us puberty occurs in its own sweet time, and while a seven- or eight-year-old girl may be wading into a sea of oestrogen, it may take a year or so of this internal bathing and development for outer changes to begin to be noticeable. At around nine to ten years old a girl's pelvic bones grow proportionally bigger, natural fat deposits begin to grow on her thighs and hips, her waist narrows, and her nipples may begin to bud. Later breast tissue and body hair (underarm, pubic and often leg and arm hair) will grow. Because girls enter puberty, usually about two years earlier than boys, girl's long-bones mature and close earlier, which is why they don't generally grow as tall as boys.

> *Mom always talked very openly about reproduction and sexuality. I had access to a whole encyclopaedia collection on reproduction and sex from age eight in my room and could look up anything I had questions about. I also read my mother's pregnancy books by the time I was ten. I have always found all of this fascinating including the ins and outs of my own cycle and bleeding.*

During puberty, fat tissue increases about a hundred and twenty-five per cent in the two years before menarche, until it averages twenty-seven per cent of a girl's total weight. It is the overall changes in the distribution of fat in the body that give rise to a girl's development of 'womanly' contours. This informs the recommended range of proportion of fat to total weight for fertile women, notwithstanding our changing understanding of weight and the influence of movements like Health At Every Size (HAES).

One of the (imperfect) rules of thumb regarding when to expect menarche is that it will occur about two years from the first signs of pubic hair, which is at first sparse and soft and in time becomes progressively longer, darker, thicker and curlier. Over time the uterus, vagina, labia, and clitoris[iii] all grow and mature, and breasts and overall body shape continue to develop according to a girl's own timing, genetics and environmental influences.

In the months before menarche many girls notice changes in their vaginal fluids, or more accurately, notice that they have them, with more profuse, wet or creamy fluid appearing from time to time on their underwear or toilet paper. Similarly, girls, and their families, often notice heightened emotional sensitivity and reactiveness. All of this is totally normal.

These are signs that the day of menarche is approaching. However, when that day will be and where it will occur all remain a mystery until it happens. Like birth stories, women's menarche stories are unique: where you were, how you felt, what you knew and what you didn't, who you told, who helped, who didn't, what you thought and whether you were celebrated, humiliated or ignored.

The first sign of blood on toilet paper, or underwear or pyjamas is usually small in quantity and reddish-brown-black in colour and may not be much in volume the first time. Of course, there are some girls who bleed profusely, and the blood is bright red straight up. Whether menarche heralds a regular period, or a year or two of a 'show' here and there, this is all within the normal range.

Even with the onset of periods the first egg may not be released for up to another couple of years, though from the outlier cases of very early pregnancies this is clearly not always the case. Once periods have begun a girl will remain fertile, all going well, until the supply of viable eggs runs out at menopause. During this fertile period of her life she will experience her menstrual cycle fairly regularly, except when she is pregnant or postpartum or using ovulation supressing contraception.

Age at menarche

There is widespread concern that the age at which girls get their first period is getting younger and younger. What's really happening here?

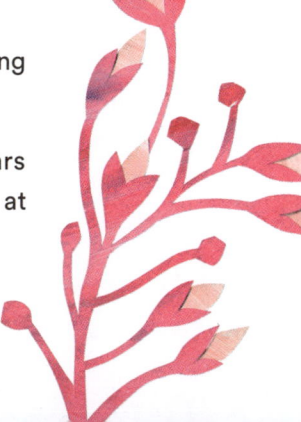

Girls in Ancient Rome started menstruating at about thirteen to fourteen years old, girls during the Early Middle Ages (400 to 1100AD) averaged fourteen years at menarche, during the Renaissance (1300 to 1600AD) they were around sixteen years and in the Victorian Era (1800s) girls were about 16.6 years in 1860, and fourteen by 1901, when they got their first period.

During the 20th century some average ages at menarche were: 13.9 in 1928 in the US, 13.5 in 1960 in the UK, and 12.8 in 1970 in the US. Girls now experience menarche around 12 to 12.7 in most developed countries.[iv]

Why are these ages so diverse?

Theories about and research into why the age at menarche has dropped in the last two centuries vary from the rise of indoor lighting impacting hormone production, presence of a nongenetically related man in the home, stress, hormones in milk and meat, increased dietary sugar, exposure to synthetic xenoestrogens, reaching a body-weight needed for menarche earlier and improved nutrition (especially animal protein). While none of these is the single cause, improved nutrition and increased animal protein are the statistical front-runners – nature's way of saying 'you're good to go', even if you are not.

That said, it's worth remembering that, rather than being on a straight downward slope, the age at which we get our first period has been all over the place throughout history. There's no such thing as too young or too old to begin because really, it's all relative and hugely variable. Clearly a girl getting her first period at ten will have quite different needs than a fifteen-year-old, and either way it's important girls are prepared and offered positive and ongoing support.

Professors Mark Hanson and Peter Gluckman researched the age of puberty stretching back beyond the Stone Age. They found that Paleolithic girls arrived at menarche between seven and thirteen years, which suggested to them that this is the evolutionarily determined age of puberty in girls.

According to Hanson and Gluckman, disease and poor nutrition became more common as humans settled, causing puberty to be delayed. Modern hygiene, nutrition and medicine have allowed the age of menarche to fall to its original range. However, today there is a mismatch between sexual maturity and psychosocial maturity, with sexual maturity occurring much earlier. This mismatch is a result of society becoming vastly more complex, with psychosocial maturity therefore taking longer to reach.

In summarising their research Professor Hanson says, 'All our social systems work on the presumption that the two types of maturity coincide. But this is no longer the case and never will be again because we cannot change biological reality. We have to work out a new set of structures – schooling, for example – to deal with this reality.'[v]

THE BIOLOGICAL INTEGRITY OF MENSTRUATION

> *It was summer, and we were cooling off at the local pool. Suddenly I had this awful pain in my belly that I'd never had before so, kind of doubled over, I made for the toilets. Once in a cubicle and sitting I saw the blood swirling around the bowl and, panicked, thought I was dying and screamed for my parents. My mum rushed in, saw what was happening and tried to calm me down, all while wadding up toilet paper to put in to my wet bathers until we got home. My dad was anxiously calling from outside just to make it all the more embarrassing and confusing.*

Adulthood: fertility

After menarche a girl is considered fertile, although it can take six to eight years for her reproductive system to fully mature. A regular cycle may take time to establish and when it does menstruation will occur twelve or so times a year to around 50 years of age.

So, in an average woman's life this is significant! She will be impacted by it physically, emotionally, psychologically, socially, financially, professionally, culturally and in terms of her religious practice, workplace, recreation, class, sexuality and reproduction.

> *I had a lot of difficulty using tampons because I had no idea how my body worked. I was doing a lot of ballet and lived away from home when my period started. My friends were long past these initial experiences and I was too embarrassed to ask them. When I was struggling to figure out tampons it was painful, I couldn't get them in properly and I was totally distracted by what was happening and worried that someone would find out. This led to some embarrassing, even humiliating experiences.*

Most women menstruate for an average of five days a month, over roughly 35 to 40 years of their life, which amounts to six or seven years of actual menstrual bleeding during 400 to 500 separate occasions. During these years, periods may cease (called amenorrhoea) for reasons including pregnancy, breastfeeding and hormonal contraception, as well as for traumatic causes like eating disorders, extreme weight loss, malnutrition, chronic or extreme stress and surgery, and medical conditions like PCOS, or intentional activities like fasting, intense physical training and crossing time zones at speed.

The average length of a menstrual cycle, from the beginning of one period to the beginning of the next is 29 to 30 days. It is interesting to note that the generally accepted 28-day norm was actually introduced by the manufacturers of the original oral contraceptive pill, to fit neat into four weeks (with the withdrawal-bleed 'period' timed for mid-week by the original male developers). So, the four-week menstrual cycle is an artificial construct and our bodies more naturally synchronise with lunar rhythms, with the average lunar cycle of 29 ½ days being closer to the average length of a menstrual cycle.[vi] That said there is great variation and women may have cycles that vary from much shorter to much longer than the norm. They may also vary greatly within a woman's individual experience, which can be of a very short cycle (such as 21 days) under some circumstances, and a rather long cycle (such as 36 days or more) at other times.

The cycling body is at any time somewhere in the ovulation-menstruation cycle, and a good understanding of this process as it repeats over months, years and decades can help a woman to *know her body, predict her moods and emotional and physical needs, have better control over her fertility and contraception, and be better able to navigate relationships, healthcare and self-care.* At any given moment, the female reproductive system is doing something important and frankly amazing, and menstruation is simply a part of that.

> *My five-year-old boy has an elementary understanding of what it means for a woman to have her period: that each month her uterus prepares a welcoming lining to see if a man's seed can find an egg to make a baby with, and if there is no baby the uterus washes the lining away. I can ask him to grab me a pad or tampon from the other bathroom and it's not a topic of shame or embarrassment for either of us. I feel good about normalizing it for him because it was a taboo source of secrecy, whispering, and shame for me when I was a girl. I believe this will help him not only to avoid toxic shame, and hopefully avoid a teen pregnancy later on. One day he'll be involved in a relationship and I want him to be like his father, to be comfortable and helpful and know what tampons or pads to buy when his girlfriend or wife sends him to the shop :)*

Once set in train at menarche, the menstrual cycle is an *ongoing cycle*, so it is imprecise to talk about how it 'starts' each month. What we can say is that the hypothalamus is in continual communication with the pituitary gland which in turn messages the ovaries, hormonally directing tasks to be completed in a set sequence. Hormones released by the ovaries also alert the hypothalamus as to what has happened and to see what needs to be done next. In this way sex hormones are produced in precise quantities and in a precise order all to maximise our fertility and chance of conception. The importance of the players in this dialogue is reflected in its rather politico-militaristic name, the HPO Axis (Hypothalamic-Pituitary-Ovarian axis).

Hormones are awesome

Since hormones were first discovered in 1902, experts in the field continue to uncover more and more about their exquisitely choreographed dance. Hormones are intrinsic to the whole human story, however for our purpose here it's female hormones that are more sharply in our focus. For those interested in exploring the male hormone story there are publications by expert authors, including Jed Diamond's cornerstone works *Male Menopause* and *The Irritable Male Syndrome*. Hormone therapy is often also important to trans and GNC people in affirming their identity.

While there is still much more to be discovered and understood, what is clear is that we need to approach our hormone-producing endocrine system with great respect.

Hormones affect how we think and feel, and how we think and feel affects our hormones. They fluctuate with our moods and emotions and have often been called 'molecules of emotion'. We know that laughter changes our hormonal responses and affects our pain threshold – for instance people with depression have very different brain-hormone patterns than those without – and that relaxation has a different hormonal profile to that of stress.

Hormones are also our body's means of connecting the external world to our internal world, sensing and responding to changes in external stimulus like temperature, safety and comfort.

Our master endocrine gland is the hypothalamus, which has been likened to the conductor of an orchestra. This gland is located deep in the brain and 'listens' for the hormonal messages coming from a person's organs, glands and tissues. It then advises the pituitary gland to send messages back to the numerous glands in the body to maintain a dynamic hormonal balance. The hypothalamus and pituitary work around the clock to synchronise our bodily functions, to help us to survive, cope with the effects of stress, assist digestion, regulate the sleep-wake cycle and support fertility. Rather wonderfully we have a specialised area in our hypothalamus called 'the menstrual clock', which has the specific job of, you guessed it, measuring and regulating the periodic timing of the menstrual cycle.

During a normal menstrual cycle, the sex hormone levels, oestrogen, progesterone, LH, FSH and testosterone fluctuate considerably. This fluctuation also causes measurable changes in most of a woman's bodily functions – including temperature, metabolism, nutritional uptake, blood sugar levels, blood acidity, heart rate, pain threshold, brain waves, the make-up of urine, the size of pupils, the sense of sight, sound and smell, the relative lumpiness and size of breasts, cervical mucus secretions and the position and relative openness of the cervix, the relative swelling of the vulva, sexual interest and sleep and energy cycles *to name just a few*. Is it any wonder that as this process repeats over and over it has such a profound effect on us?

> Having a baby and now trying for a second baby makes me appreciate my periods more - I am very in tune with my cycles, where I am in the month and how I'm feeling. I'm much **more connected to my body** and I respect menstruation and all that comes with it because of pregnancy, birth and trying to conceive.

The cycle 'begins'

For ease of comparison and understanding we generally measure the length of a menstrual cycle from the first day of blood flow, not spotting, and call it Day 1, adding numbers a day at a time until the day before Day 1 of the next menstrual period. Using this measure menstruation is on Days 1 to 5, or thereabouts, of the menstrual cycle.

> *Having a baby and now trying for a second baby makes me appreciate my periods more — I am very in tune with my cycles, where I am in the month and how I'm feeling. I'm much more connected to my body and I respect menstruation and all that comes with it because of pregnancy, birth and trying to conceive.*

Menstruation will begin close to fourteen days after ovulation, but ovulation does not necessarily occur fourteen days after the beginning of the last period, unless a woman has a super regular 28-day cycle, and most don't.[vii] The most changeable part of the cycle is menstruation to ovulation, shrinking in a short cycle or stretching in a long one. However, the time from ovulation to menstruation is relatively stable, and when a woman knows how long this is for her, somewhere between thirteen to fifteen days, this will be consistent for her fertile life. This highlights the value of learning what should be a key life skill — being able to recognise the signs of ovulation.

> *During my 30s as we were planning to start a family, I charted my cycles and became so aware of my body. I found it really powerful to understand what was happening, and to use that information to help conceive a baby.*

The lining of the womb, the endometrium, grows from its thinnest just after menstruation to ten times that thickness at its peak, just before menstruation. By the beginning of menstruation, the uterus can be twice the weight it was after the last period, which explains, in part, the heavy dragging feeling many women report just before and early in their period as the much heavier organ pulls on its support ligaments. Shaped like a perfect pear or avocado with a little bend at its narrow end and positioned neck down in our body, the uterus is a muscular, 'hollow' organ about seven and a half centimetres long and holds about a teaspoon of liquid in its non-pregnant and non-menstruating states. In around twenty per cent of women the bulb of the uterus tilts back, in most it sits upright, and a rare woman may find she has two uteruses and two vaginas – we are nothing if not diverse. Then, when a foetus is full term, the uterus stretches up to 500 times its non-pregnant state.

Once it is clear that no fertilised egg has made its way to the uterus the temporary endocrine gland on the ovarian wall ceases its production of progesterone. This triggers the blood supply to the womb's lining via tiny corkscrew capillaries to stop, then they open again and blood floods through, effectively washing away the lining with blood. As well as this blood, menstrual fluid also contains the remains of the uterine lining, egg cells, oestrogenic hormones, lecithins, arsenic compounds and a rich concentration of essential minerals, such as iron and phosphorous, along with hitch-hiking cervical and vaginal secretions. No wonder some women (now and throughout history) like to make use of this rich mix by saving water from soaking cloth pads or diluting menstrual blood collected in a menstrual cup, to feed herbs, vegetables and other treasured plants. Menses may well have contributed to the survival of previous generations, even outside of its reproductive purpose!

So, when we notice blood in our underwear or on toilet paper the lining of the uterus has already been shed. Around two-thirds of menstrual blood is reabsorbed by the body and the rest trickles slowly over several days through the tiny softened opening of the cervix, the beautifully named 'os' at the neck of the womb. Though some days it may not feel like a gentle trickle. On a reverse journey sperm gain entry to the uterus via the os on their way to find an egg.

By volume menstrual blood is usually around two to three tablespoons, or a small medicine cup's worth, over a period's duration, although most menstruating woman will swear it is more, and for some it can truly be much, much more.

Menstrual blood may yet prove to offer benefits beyond the monthly clear-out, being an excellent plant fertiliser, and a cervical and vaginal swab (more on that later). Scientists have found that stem cells can be obtained from women's menstrual blood. These have the capacity to differentiate into heart, nerve, bone, cartilage and fat cells. Researchers have so far found that menstrual blood may be a promising source of adult stem cells for applications in regenerative medicine.[viii] Definitely a research thread to keep our eye on.

Feeling follicular

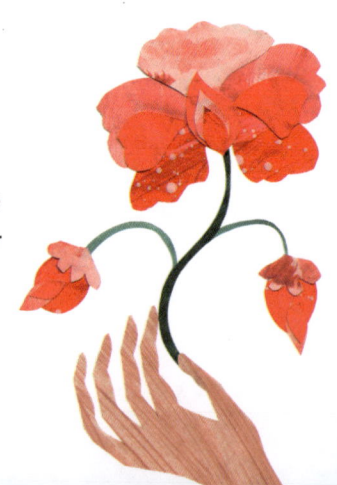

Generally, after menstruation but sometimes while still bleeding in a short cycle, the hypothalamus signals the pituitary to send FSH to the ovaries to prepare an egg for ovulation. In fact, around twenty eggs start this process each cycle although it is mostly just one that makes it through to ovulation. This is called the follicular phase and occurs between menstruation and ovulation.

When FSH reaches the ovary, it stimulates the follicles to ripen eggs, which have been prepping for their chance at ovulation for the past three months (from immature seed cell to mature egg at ovulation is one hundred days). The developing follicles in turn release oestrogen and as these levels rise during this phase it causes several important things to occur.

The first is that the cervix softens and rises, and the os widens at ovulation, all the better to welcome any visiting sperm.

Secondly, the mucus produced by mucous membranes in the cervical crypts changes in quantity and quality and becomes supportive, rather than hostile, to sperm for several days before ovulation. This protects them from the natural acidity of the vagina, ensures their life for three to six days and helps to channel and nourish them on their journey through the reproductive tract. Women often notice the greater quantity and changed quality of cervical mucus at the mouth of the vagina, or on underwear or toilet paper around this time.

> *I was uncomfortable discussing female body functions until I reached university and became best friends with a very open girl. She encouraged me to look at my body as 'no big deal', really rather fascinating and certainly nothing to be ashamed or awkward about.*

Importantly, although anatomically an extension of the uterine muscle, the cervix is an organ in its own right. It has the capacity to produce an array of mucus for specific and varied purposes, offer sperm crucial supports and protection in its crypts, and during childbirth it thins and dilates to about ten centimetres in diameter to allow the baby passage down into the vagina before closing tight again over the following weeks.

The os of a woman who has not given vaginal birth looks like a small dot in the centre of a moist, plump doughnut, whereas the os of a woman who has is thereafter stretched to a line, like an emoji representing a degree of ambivalence or perhaps a slight grimace!

Finally, the result of rising oestrogen levels is that the lining of the womb thickens and prepares to receive a possible fertilised egg. And, while there are many secondary effects of oestrogen, in general, many women find their physical energy, zest and sexual interest rises, peaking around ovulation, which makes perfect biological and evolutionary sense!

With stress, as mentioned above, the follicular phase can become shortened or lengthened, in other words, ovulation can be brought forward or delayed. Delay, leading to longer cycles, is more common and may be caused by any number of factors, including stress, travel, ill health, some medicines, excessive exercise, weight changes, diet changes, fasting or any other atypical activity. This is because of the effect these stressful events or conditions have on the fine-tuned interaction of hormones.

Ovulation: the power moment

Ovulation is truly nature's big purpose for the whole cycle, even though it all happens deep within the pelvic cavity, and outside most women's awareness.

Let's take a moment to look more closely at ovaries. These are our primary female reproductive organs and are about the size and shape of an olive or shell-bound almond, whitish in colour, and contain at birth all the (immature) eggs, or ova, that will mature and be released during a woman's fertile life, as well as hundreds of thousands of spares! As well as producing eggs ovaries are the primary producers of oestrogen and progesterone during a woman's cycling life.

> *Despite the difficulties with my period, I have treasured my cycle throughout my life as a source of deep feminine wisdom, and as one of the many rhythms of nature that bring to life a 'terrible beauty.'*

A few days before ovulation, the hypothalamus recognises the peak FSH levels indicating the eggs are now mature and instructs the pituitary gland to send a whoosh of LH, which triggers the ripest and most beautiful ova to pop out of its follicle, the bubble nurturing the egg to maturity on the outer wall of the ovary. Oestrogen is produced by ovarian follicles right through the menstrual month, and as the follicles get larger and stronger, more oestrogen is produced. As these levels increase, the lining of the uterus thickens further and after a peak at ovulation oestrogen dips precipitously, rapidly 'drying' cervical mucus production. Testosterone, though much less prolific, surges and then dips right around ovulation too.

The many works of ovulation

Researchers have found the rising levels of oestrogen and testosterone in the few days leading to ovulation coincide with shinier hair, a sweeter genital smell and taste, clearer eyes, a desire to expose more skin and, for heterosexual women, more interest in more typically 'masculine' pictures of men. Of course, there are a great many factors both environmental and personal that influence how a woman will feel on a particular day, and who she may or may not be attracted to sexually. That said it is highly conceivable that this stage of the menstrual cycle does have an effect on a woman's libido, as is frequently reported anecdotally by women.

In a study of exotic dancers and their daily tips, it was found that while performing presumably the same moves in the same costumes, their tips peaked at ovulation and remained at a steady lower level for the rest of the cycle. For those who were on the Pill their tips remained constant at the lower level. [ix]

While the biological foundations and reproductive imperative of these results are easy to see, what does this mean for women generally? For a start it is worth a woman observing her own cycle, and, if she finds there is a pattern, she can consider how she can use this as a mitigating factor in how she works with her calendar.

> *Mom was incredibly open and positive about my period and all the changes that were happening to my body. Because of her wonderful attitude I had no fear of menstruation when it arrived, and now, although I have incredibly painful cramps and severe bloating, I still feel a reverence towards my cycle. As far as possible I take it slow for one to three days of my period and get massage and acupuncture when I can.*

For some women ovulation is accompanied by a dull ache low in the abdomen that can last a few hours. This is often called by its German name, *Mittelschmerz*, which means 'middle pain'.

After ovulation the egg is greeted by the waving fronds of the nearest fallopian tube that delicately waft it into its passage. These are about seven to twelve centimetres in length, 0.5 to 1.2 centimetres in diameter and muscular, and have tendrils on their ends called fimbriae, which sweep the egg up into the tube. At this stage the mature egg is the largest single cell in the human body, and though tiny, is visible to the naked eye (about the size of the full stop at the end of this sentence) and the only human cell that is perfectly round.

The luscious luteal

If there is no waiting swarm of sperm in the fallopian tube and none arrive soon after, our hero the egg will wait eight to twenty-four hours, then calls it quits, dissolving into her components to be reabsorbed by the body. At the same time the empty follicle on the surface of the ovary becomes a temporary gland, the corpus luteum (Latin for 'yellow body'), which gives this phase of the menstrual cycle its name: the luteal phase.

The corpus luteum acts as a tiny, temporary endocrine gland that will produce progesterone (the hormone of pro-gestation, or pregnancy) until menstruation, sending signals to the lining of the uterus to ask it to thicken, ripen and prepare itself for pregnancy. If conception does take place, this gland supports the early days of pregnancy until the placenta is big enough to take over the job. After a week or so, if the uterus detects no burrowing into its rich lining by a tiny multi-cell blastocyst ball, it too will begin a hormonal signal-loop with the HPO Axis and prepare to shed its lining as surplus to requirements.

During the luteal phase the ovary continues to release oestrogen, but in reduced amounts, causing the cervix to lower, harden and close, and the mucus to become less welcoming, even hostile, to sperm.

At the same time rising progesterone levels cause the following things to occur: the body-at-rest temperature rises, the uterine lining thickens even more, so that within five to seven days it is ready to welcome a fertilised egg, fully supplied with blood and nutrients.

The lifespan of the corpus luteum is about twelve to sixteen days, and it does not vary much, either from woman to woman or cycle to cycle. So, menstruation is nearly always about two weeks after the preceding ovulation, and not, as sometimes mistakenly thought, reliably two weeks before the next.

All the while, the hypothalamus and pituitary are listening to these hormonal messages via feedback. If the egg is not fertilised, the hypothalamus and pituitary gland direct the corpus luteum to discontinue hormone production, resulting in a drop in progesterone levels that then triggers the uterine lining to shed and join the menstrual flow. The corpus luteum shrivels to a tiny white scar on the surface of the ovary, the corpus albicans (Latin for 'white body').

> I wish I'd **understood my cycle** from a much earlier age. When I was learning about natural contraception in my mid-twenties, it astounded me that I'd been menstruating for over a decade and not been taught to really understand what was happening. Knowing the times when I was fertile and when I wasn't gave me a **deep appreciation of my power** to choose whether and when I wanted to conceive. This knowledge really did feel like a special female super power.

Owner's Manual: reading the signs of your fertility

At the risk of restating the obvious, a woman's fertility is cyclic in nature and goes through constant change. By learning to read these changes we can understand what these signs and symptoms mean, know where we are in our cycle, and even what we can do to manage symptoms of cyclic imbalance.

> *I wish I'd understood my cycle from a much earlier age. When I was learning about natural contraception in my mid-twenties, it astounded me that I'd been menstruating for over a decade and not been taught to really understand what was happening. Knowing the times when I was fertile and when I wasn't gave me a deep appreciation of my power to choose whether and when I wanted to conceive. This knowledge really did feel like a special female super power.*

While most of us may not be so attuned to our finely orchestrated menstrual cycle, this may in part be because it simply hasn't been suggested to us. Medical science is, after all, only just beginning to research the benefits of the menstrual cycle for women.[x]

The most obvious and unmistakable sign of your fertility cycle is the arrival of your period every month. You can learn to recognise numerous other signs as you observe certain regular predictable patterns. There are lots of benefits of getting to know your cycle, including knowing when your period is due, understanding the different stages, reducing or eliminating menstrual problems, understanding your cyclic emotions, planning with your energy levels in mind and managing your fertility itself.

In order to get to know your cycle better you may like to chart various signs over several months. Here are the important concepts to grasp first.

Temperature

As mentioned, after ovulation the follicle that released the mature egg becomes a temporary endocrine gland, the corpus luteum, and produces progesterone. Among other effects of increased progesterone your temperature will rise, so from ovulation to menstruation, your basal, or body-at-rest, temperature will be several tenths of a degree higher. By taking your temperature every morning before rising and marking this on a chart (or app) you will start to see the pattern of your own cycle emerging. Most commonly this will be a chart with two temperature phases, one phase before ovulation and a phase of higher temperature after. If pregnancy takes place the chart becomes tri-phasic and the temperature goes up even further once the endometrium registers the presence of a zygote. For many women this is the first discernible proof of pregnancy.

A chart that shows no significant shift in temperature, other than small daily variations, indicates an anovulatory cycle, that is one where there are sufficient hormones for the cycle to end in a bleed, but in which no ovulation has taken place. This is quite common, especially early and late in a woman's cycling career.

Cervical mucus

Mucus, the product of the mucous membranes of the cervix, changes significantly in texture, colour and quantity during your cycle. This mucus is rich in antiseptic enzymes, immunoglobulins, inorganic salts, proteins, glycoproteins and water. However, the observable features will vary somewhat from girl to girl and woman to woman, and it is useful to get to know your own pattern. To check your mucus gently collect some on your middle or pointer finger at the opening of your vagina before you urinate. Lightly touch your finger and thumb together and notice the texture of the mucus. How would you describe this to yourself?

The mucus produced in the crypts of the cervix flows toward the opening of the vagina. Collected there and observed this can tell you a great deal about your cyclic fertility and your reproductive, hormonal and even general health.

Generally, the first mucus you will notice after menstruation will be opaque, thick, dry, flaky and crumbly and it will hold its shape when pressed. It will be unchanging in quantity. This is Infertile Mucus. After some days, or a week or so, this will change to more damp, pasty and tacky and increase in quantity. This is Probably Infertile Mucus. Several days before ovulation this will change to translucent, milky-white or pink, thin, wet, fluid, creamy and slippery and will be of increasing amounts. This is Fertile Mucus. For many, but not all, girls and women, their mucus will then turn stretchy, like raw egg-white, and be profuse in quantity. This is Extremely Fertile Mucus. The last day of either Fertile or Extremely Fertile Mucus signals the day before ovulation (for 85% of women), or two days before ovulation (for 10% of women).

We can easily imagine women in many parts of the world, over the many tens of thousands of years of human existence, noticing changes in the fluids emerging from their vagina (and not just blood) alongside the manifold changes noticed in nature around them. After noticing these patterns, it is also easy to imagine this wisdom being passed on to girls and young women with each generation.

An Aboriginal elder, Niranji, in Victoria reported to Dr. Evelyn Billings [xi] that traditionally when Wurundjeri girls started to menstruate they were taken away to a sacred place by older women and taught how to recognise the different types of mucus present at different stages of their cycle. It is also known that at least three African tribal groups (the Taita, Kamba and Luo) have taught girls about the changes in mucus produced by the cervix as a marker of fertility generations past. [xii]

There are stories of First Nations women of North America using smooth river stones as tools for understanding their fertility. The river stones were passed gently over the labia to identify the presence of fertile and infertile mucus. With fertile mucus the stone would glide smoothly, and with the thicker and less prolific infertile mucus it would find resistance. [xiii] This practice would often take place at dusk, as part of an evening ritual, and it's easy to see the benefits these women would have gained, by building this intimacy with themselves and their bodies, as well as a healthy self-awareness.

When women have had some experience observing and charting their cervical mucus this awareness becomes second nature, like knowing whether they are hungry or thirsty or tired. A World Health Organization (WHO) survey in five developing countries showed that over 90% of women were able to return an interpretable chart of their cervical mucus changes by the end of the first cycle, and equally so for women who had had no formal education. Clearly, learning to understand changes in cervical mucus is something almost all cycling girls and women can do with great benefit.

While testing oestrogen levels to detect ovulation at Edinburgh University Professor John Brown found 'women's own awareness of their cervical mucus could indicate ovulation even more accurately than direct measurement of oestrogen.' [xiv] There are numerous other observable signs of fertility, like position and texture of the cervix, relative swelling of the vulva and alternate swelling of the inguinal lymph nodes at ovulation (found deep in the crease where the thigh and trunk meet), indicating whether it was the left or right ovary which ovulated, which all going well, should alternate).

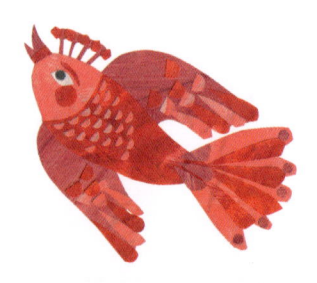

Viva la vulva

In recent years the term 'vagina' has often been used to describe the whole genital area. As a colloquial cultural flowering, in large part aimed at practicing and spreading comfort in saying, hearing and seeing the word vagina, that's fine. However, it isn't anatomically correct and results in many women and girls being unclear about what's what. So, let's have a brief genital review here.

The external genitalia are collectively called the vulva and are separated from the anus by the perineum. The genitals include the mons pubis, clitoris, the inner and outer labia, the urethral and vaginal openings. Just like any other part of the body, vulvae vary enormously and come in all shapes, sizes and colours. Many women have never seen their own due to the need to be either very bendy or sufficiently comfortable to have a look. We can't overstate how important it is to do this if you can! Sit in front of a large mirror, or hold a small one, to get to know this important and powerful part of your body. Your sex life, your sexual health, your childbirth experience, and yes, your menstruation and menopause could all be seriously improved as a result!

The inner lips, the labia minora in Latin, together with the outer lips, the labia majora, are the soft folds of skin that protect the vaginal opening. The majora are plumper than the minora and sport their own special short and curly hair. Labia come in all shapes, sizes, colours and textures.

Pubic hair is the hair that grows around the genital and anal regions. It also varies in colour, texture, length and thickness and often extends up the front or back or onto the thighs and is generally darker and curlier than hair elsewhere on the body. Pubic hair provides protection and cushioning to the genitals and protects against infection. It also transmits sensation and does important work capturing scent and pheromones. The urethra, which is just in front of the vaginal opening is the tiny outer opening for the bladder – in other words where we urinate from.

The opening of the vagina is between the urethra and the dense musculature of the perineum. The vagina itself is the internal passage about ten to fifteen centimetres long that connects the uterus with the outside world. It is a uniquely muscular organ that expands during sexual arousal, and during birth, when it becomes engorged with blood and secretes a lubricating fluid. It contracts, along with the uterine muscles, during orgasm, which, as many would agree, is an important function!

Just below where the labia minora meet is the outer visible part of the clitoris. The clitoris contains 15,000 nerve endings, with the tip of the clitoris (the glans) usually the most sensitive area of the vulva. This exquisite sensitivity is protected by the prepuce, or hood of the clitoris. The clitoris fills with blood, and becomes firm and erect, like a penis, during arousal. They are, after all, formed from the same foetal tissue. The clitoris is the only organ in the entire body that has the sole purpose of sexual arousal or pleasure.

Incredibly the clitoris was only fully mapped in the 1990s by Dr Helen O'Connell from the University of Melbourne (formerly Melbourne University), when she showed us that the clitoris is actually much bigger than previously understood. Once thought to be just the little round glans and hood that are visible we now know there are legs (crura) and bulbs that extend to either side of the vaginal opening. Thank you, Helen!

In honour of the vulva and its metaphorical and actual importance carvings of a naked woman spreading her legs to display an exaggerated vulva, Sheela na Gig figures, were produced between the 12th and 17th centuries in Great Britain and Ireland and can be found in abundance above the portals of churches and castles there. These are quite possibly based on much older pre-Christian fertility symbols. Maybe we need more vulvae carved in to buildings now!

A vagina by another name may be understood and respected differently

Leah Kaminsky, a Melbourne novelist and doctor, recently wrote 'The case for renaming women's body parts' for the BBC.[xv] She explored the whys and wherefores of the naming and describing of many female body parts and conditions after male doctors, and how this legacy skews our perceptions of women's bodies.

'Hysteria' comes from the Greek word for uterus, 'hysterika', and was described by Hippocrates as the condition caused by a wandering uterus. The cure for a wandering uterus was thought to be marriage and lots of sex (consensual or otherwise). It was only in 1952 that the American Psychiatric Association finally removed 'hysteria' from their list of modern diseases.

Examples of naming body parts are: the Pouch of Douglas (James Douglas) is tucked behind the uterus, Bartholin's Glands (Caspar Bartholin) open into the vagina and produce a thin mucus to lubricate the vagina, fallopian tubes (Gabriel Fallopian) gather up mature eggs at one end and deposit a fertilised egg, or perhaps the remains of an unfertilised one, into the uterus at the other, and the erogenous G spot (Ernst Gräfenberg) located on the front wall of the vagina. As an aside, the G-spot is now thought to be the position where the internal part of the clitoris passes next to the vaginal wall.

Perhaps most telling of all is the origin of 'vagina', derived from the Latin word for sheath or scabbard and named such in the late 17th century. Clearly referring to its sometimes relationship to the penis the word vagina suggests that the rest of the time it is merely a 'scabbard' in waiting. So we use a word for women's genitals that literally implies it's a receptacle for a penis. Not ideal!

While it is not surprising that in a patriarchy female body parts are named from a male perspective, as we become more conscious of gender equity issues and work to address them this is certainly one of the many territories that needs serious attention. As Lera Boroditsky, Associate Professor of Cognitive Science at the University of California San Diego says, these terms should be replaced by descriptors that are useful and educational to the body's owner.

We agree wholeheartedly. And simultaneously, while new terms are being conceived, recognise the value of using the current imperfect but known terms that we already have for the important work of supporting women and girls to understand their own bodies and thereby to have greater agency. Ideally these projects will progress together and be closely aware of each other.

> *I spent so many years railing against my female body. It took so long to gain a proper acceptance of being in this body but even now I still count myself as being on the transgender spectrum. It'll be interesting, after menopause finally happens, to see just where my feelings on gender settle.*

A delightful example of thoughtful introduction of a new word is the story of Anna Kostztovics, a Swedish social worker who was concerned about the ramifications of girls not having a non-sexualised word for their genitals, whereas boys did, 'snoop', a common term roughly like the English 'willy'. Kostztovics went on to popularise a new friendly, non-sexualised word as the female equivalent, 'snippa'. Lovely!

Trans and GNC people are also leading thoughtful conversations about how we refer to body parts and systems, in liberating and revolutionary ways.

Menstrual mathematics

With all the adding, subtracting and counting cycle after cycle it is no wonder that a number of scholars have linked women tracking their menstrual cycle with the early development of mathematics and calendars.

Mathematician John Kellermeier has found that menstruation played a key role in the development of counting and measuring time through anthropological artifacts.[xvi]

Many other scholars also assert that women invented timekeeping through charting their menses on various animal bones and beads. For instance, the Lebombo Bone (35,000BC), the oldest mathematical instrument to be discovered, is a baboon fibula and has 29 distinct markings, which are thought to have been used to track menstrual or lunar cycles or, quite possibly, both at once.[xvii]

Women's menstrual awareness has also played a major role in the early development of calendars, with Romans calling the calculation of time mensuration, i.e. knowledge of the menses. In Latin *mensura* is measurement, and *menstrua* is a grammatical form of menstrous or monthly. The Gaelic word for 'menstruation' and 'calendar' is similarly identical.[xviii]

But why, oh why do we menstruate?

The answer to this question is an evolving one, with numerous pieces of the puzzle at hand, and undoubtedly more yet to be uncovered. Here's what we do know.

Most mammals don't menstruate, but instead build up a thickened endometrium if fertilisation occurs. However, most primates, which includes lemurs, monkeys, apes, lorises, a few bats, elephant shrews, and humans, do.

Some partial explanations for the occurrence of menstruation in those of us who do are:

- that menstruation flushes out pathogens, which enter the reproductive tract having hitched a ride on sperm, *but that phenomenon is ubiquitous so why do just a few species bother with menstruation?* Maybe this is just a happy side-benefit not a cause; and

- that it's more efficient to flush out the thickened endometrium when we don't need it in terms of the nutrition and the energy needed to maintain it constantly, *estimated to be a day and half of extra food a month.* Yes, but most mammals' endometrium only builds for fertilisation anyway. Still, this makes economic sense for us.

In 2012, biologist Deena Emera and her team from Yale University published their findings on the evolution of menstruation in *Bioessays*.[xix]

The answer to the question of menstruation suggested by Emera and her crew is that it is purely evolutionary and involves maternal-foetal conflict and concurrent conflict between the father's genes and the mother's ongoing reproductive interests. *What does all that mean?*

Emera's theory is that a process called *decidualisation*, or the production of a thickened lining of the uterus, is the key, not menstruation.

In most mammals decidualisation occurs *in response* to fertilisation, when the thickening of the endometrium, or decidualisation, only occurs once the lining receives the chemical signal from the embryo saying, 'I'm here, please make my bed!'.

In a few, including us and most primates, decidualisation occurs spontaneously and regularly, whether or not there is a fertilised embryo.

Among mammals there is variation between how deeply the placenta attaches itself to the uterus: superficially, deeper into the uterine lining, and deeper still into the maternal blood vessels, which is described as hemochorial. *All mammalian species that menstruate are hemochorial.* Bingo!

In species like us with especially 'invasive' placentas we need to build up a thicker and more protective endometrium pre-emptively, before and in case of fertilisation.

Then, *if fertilisation does not occur*, the hormone progesterone responsible for maintaining the lining declines, so the lining is shed, and menstruation occurs.

If fertilisation does occur the prepared lining is more able to detect foetal quality and abort early if it is not viable. Women vary in their degree of decidualisation, some who have reduced decidualisation capacity may get pregnant more easily, but also have pregnancy loss more often too.

So, the biological battle between foetus, father and mother goes like this: the foetus is genetically primed to *survive at all costs* and the father's reproductive interests are to have his genes propagated *in any one pregnancy*; however, for the mother, if conditions are not optimal in any one pregnancy, it is in the woman's reproductive interests to bail out and try again another time. *Phew!*

From the work of Emera and her colleagues we can see that it is likely that somewhere along the human evolutionary path, the dialogue between embryo and uterus shifted, so that the signals causing the endometrium to thicken came not from the embryo, but from the mother herself. Instead of being linked to the presence of the embryo, uterine thickening became linked to ovulation and the choreographed hormones that each woman cycles through on a monthly basis.

So, that is the best we can do on the *Why?* question for now. Look out for further developments on this.

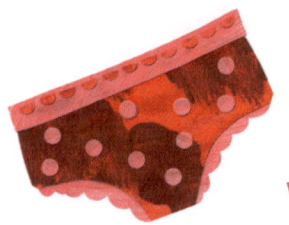

What if menstruation was optional?

In Australia and other countries, we are seeing a trend towards menstrual suppression, the artificial elimination of the menstrual cycle, using synthetic hormones in the form of either oral contraceptives, or implants, injections or patches. This off-label use of contraceptives is often not related to reproductive health but is rather specifically to prevent ovulation and menstruation from occurring altogether.

This cultural shift is partly enabled by the perception of hormonal contraception as 'neutral' and not medical; the Pill is seen as somehow different to other pharmaceutical drugs, with women who take it sometimes forgetting to disclose it in medical situations where they are asked if they are currently on any prescription drugs. The other decisive factor in how women have embraced the idea of not having a period at all is the power of the menstrual taboo, which teaches girls and women that periods not only have no value but are disgusting, taxing and unnecessary. The obvious exception to this is the number of women suffering menstrual dysfunction who turn to menstrual suppression as a treatment, in order to reduce pain or incapacitation each month, while they work towards a diagnosis or in some cases, surgical intervention. That said, increasing numbers of perfectly healthy women are opting to simply 'cancel' their period, and this requires some examination.

So who recommends menstrual suppression? More and more, it's other women. Word of mouth accounts for a large reason why the practice has spread, including the sharing of stories online as well as offline. But women can't prescribe these medications to each other, so who else thinks it's a good idea? Doctors, obviously, are in some cases suggesting these drugs, but also responding to patient requests. So where did the idea come from? Partly, it was women as well – for many years, women have skipped the placebo pills and missed their periods anyway. Now pharmaceutical companies have developed long-acting reversible contraceptives (LARCs) and new versions of the Pill marketed with this specific goal in mind. Drug manufacturers have significant influence on doctors' education and prescribing habits and reinforce this through advertising campaigns.

Some scientists have come out strongly in favour of menstrual suppression too, none more so than Elsimar Coutinho, the Brazilian gynaecologist and one of the developers of the injectable LARC, Depo Provera. In 1999, he published a book called *Is Menstruation Obsolete? How suppressing menstruation can help women who suffer from anaemia, endometriosis, or PMS* in which he argues strongly in favour of women dispensing with menstruation altogether. The book attracted widespread criticism from women's health professors and practitioners, for its basic premise, methodology and rigour, but it also became a pop cultural curiosity, picked up in a mainstream media hungry for medico-scientific narratives and sensational stories. Coutinho argues that because prehistoric women had far fewer periods in the course of a lifetime, because they spent more time pregnant and breastfeeding, it is unnatural, unnecessary and even dangerous for women to menstruate so often. It's one of those arguments with the ring of logic, but actually runs counter to the evidence we do have that women have always used contraception to manage their reproductive destinies, in one form or another, whereas Coutinho lacks a strong anthropological basis for his claims. It is also flawed logic to suggest that taking synthetic hormones brings about a more 'natural' state for women and their bodies, than what their bodies actually naturally do.

Much critique of menstrual suppression centres on the fact that we just do not know enough about the long-term effects of these drugs: on fertility, on the overall health of the body, on the women who use them. The Pill has been through serious revisions and recalibrations since its inception, partly due to emerging evidence of its negative health impacts. Another cautionary tale exists in the widespread promotion and prescription of Hormone Replacement Therapy (HRT) for menopausal symptoms. Decades after it became popular in the 1960s, research released in the 1990s proved that HRT was associated with elevated risk of breast cancer, heart disease and osteoporosis. While subsequent research has added complexity to these findings, the fact remains that large-scale use of medications before we know of the health risks is logically to be avoided, especially when they are prescribed to healthy women. Just as the Pill is prescribed to healthy girls and women once they reach a certain age, as a precautionary measure against unwanted pregnancy and increasingly off-label, so too HRT is often taken up by women as a pre-emptive strike against the symptoms of menopause.

Endocrinology is such a young branch of medicine, especially in terms of what we simply do not know about the production and behaviour of hormones. But gaining approval by the Food and Drug Administration (FDA) in the USA, or the Therapeutic Goods Association (TGA) in Australia, does not correlate directly to the safety of a drug. What these agencies regulate is whether or not companies *properly disclose* possible side effects, which is very different to deciding whether or not a medication is safe, especially when used for off-label purposes. The emerging practice wisdom of experts in the fields of fertility and women's health paints a different picture, where practitioners are increasingly questioning the assertion of pharmaceutical companies that there is no connection between birth control use and fertility (more specifically, subsequent optimum conditions for conception), when their clinical experience says otherwise.

In the case of hormonal contraception, there are serious ethical concerns cutting across the debate, including the widespread prescription of LARCs to communities like Indigenous girls and disabled women. This is a continuation of the problematic inception of the Pill itself, which has always been of interest to those invested in corrupt ideas like eugenics, white supremacy and ableism. Adolescent girls across society are keen adopters of menstrual suppression, and even some supporters of the practice warn against this. The fact is that the menstrual cycle produces hormones that are conducive to our overall health. Completely doing away with it, even in the case of menstrual dysfunction, can have deleterious long-term effects, even though it's clear why some seek the relief they do. Much more research is needed to know exactly what the price is that we are being asked to pay.

This is the unavoidable truth: reproductive rights, and the medical interventions we develop to guarantee them, how they are developed and sold, and for what reason, is highly complex terrain. The tendency towards totalising answers, as well as the power of negative attitudes toward menstruation, often obscures this. Arguing that any particular path is the right one for all women is not only irresponsible, but it's also guaranteed to fail. Each body is different and needs its own plan. Women deserve to have the agency that can only come from informed choice and this requires nuance. There are no easy answers but first we need to be asking the right questions. We'll explore this further in A Pervasive Menstrual Taboo.

Period troubles

So, what about menstrual problems? Headaches, migraine, nausea, sore breasts, bloating, acne, fatigue, mood-swings, depression, irritability? Endometriosis, Polycystic ovarian syndrome, fibroids, painful and heavy periods by other causes, premenstrual syndrome and premenstrual dysphoric disorder? Normal, treatable or just part of the deal?

While many menstrual problems are triggered or exacerbated by hormonal imbalance, they can also be heightened by conditions that are especially symptomatic at certain times in the menstrual cycle but not otherwise related to fertility, like diabetes and bipolar disorder.

> *I wish I had been offered treatment much earlier in my life. What a different kind of life I could have had. I have had three miscarriages that were very traumatic, and I sometimes have PTSD (Post Traumatic Stress Disorder) episodes triggered by excessive bleeding. I can't talk to anyone about this easily or openly and I go through hell trying to stop thinking about the miscarriages while I'm menstruating.*

Most women intuitively sense the difference between hormonal health and imbalance, and what imbalance feels like. When our hormones are 'all over the place' this can lead to an array of health problems as well as emotional distress.

The hormones that perform the intricate communication loops in our body do so in exquisitely small quantities. Oestradiol, for instance, is measured in parts per trillion. Imagine a drop of gin in sixty train tanks of tonic. A part per trillion. In these concentrations hormonal balance is clearly highly vulnerable to the stressors that can throw it out and the menstrual cycle is the proverbial canary in the coalmine. When we have period problems we are warned that all is not well.

Let's think about it like this: the menstrual cycle itself is not a disease. In fact, our fertility is an explicit sign of our health and wellbeing, and of itself is normal and healthy for women between the ages of ten and sixty, give or take (except for the equally normal and healthy state of pregnancy, post-natal amenorrhoea and menopause).

The key hormones known to upset the delicate balance of the menstrual cycle are prolactin and cortisol. Prolactin is produced in the pituitary gland and should be released in only very low levels through the cycle. However, in the event of excessive or chronic stress (emotional, environmental, physical, nutritional, biological), prolactin is over stimulated by the stress hormone cortisol. Research has linked elevated prolactin to PMS, PCOS, delayed ovulation, heavy periods, infertility and low progesterone levels (which itself leads to conditions of oestrogen dominance). Considering elevated prolactin is a result of elevated cortisol (most commonly), what really tips the balance is stress. Your emotional experiences, no matter how big or small, have a profound impact on your hormonal and cyclic health. Our body recognises stress as elevations of cortisol and decreased levels of the protective, anti-aging longevity hormone DHEA (dehydroepiandrosterone). Not only has elevated cortisol been linked to female hormone imbalances, it is also closely associated with immune suppression (especially natural killer cells, which are responsible for cancer prevention), osteoporosis, hypertension, anxiety and insomnia.

Simply put, survival trumps reproduction, so that you can live to procreate another day. With limited base material the hormone progesterone can be co-opted to make cortisol to cope with stress, which is great as it can help us do what we need to do to survive. However, if stress is chronic and our sex hormones are constantly being pulled from their own task to help with another, chronic imbalance is the inevitable result. When our cyclic hormones become unbalanced, we start to experience symptoms.

All those symptoms we feel – the bloating and mood swings, heavy bleeding and painful cramps or at peri-menopause the hot flushes and foggy brain – these are all signs of hormonal imbalance.

So, when we begin to experience symptoms, instead of blaming our hormones, here's what we need to know: our hormonal messengers telling us about these imbalances will get louder and louder until we learn to listen – it is stress that turns 'hormones' into symptoms. It is not the hormones themselves that are the problem.

When we 'develop' symptoms, it's not like developing an illness or catching a virus. That's why 'treating' them without tending to the stressors in our lives will not work past suppressing symptoms temporarily, not that anyone can be blamed for wanting that.

Consequently, rather than think of the menstrual cycle as the culprit, and it's easy to see why many of us do, it can in fact be a very helpful health assessment tool, especially for women who have some familiarity with what the normal signs of fertility should be. For this reason, some women's-health medical specialists, as noted, are beginning to recommend to their colleagues to consider the menstrual cycle as a vital sign, the observation of which can give very useful information about overall health, possible disease states and avenues for restoring wellbeing.

With an appreciative eye we can see that the menstrual cycle, and the precise and changing menu of hormone cocktails women are bathed in daily, provides us with a unique feedback loop that gives us detailed information about how we are travelling both physically and psychologically. If we are overly or chronically stressed in our work, home life or relationships, if our diet is dodgy over an extended period, if we have a reproductive or other health condition, these will often show up as symptoms premenstrually and menstrually. Commonly we bemoan our period for this discomfort, but with a minor change of lens we may see that in fact the fluctuations of the menstrual cycle offer us an opportunity to see, and by seeing to act.

Then, just as we are starting to get the hang of it all, it changes again.

When periods start to stop

Peri-menopause is the term that refers to the years leading to menopause. Prolific women's health author Dr Christiane Northrup calls this time 'the mother of all wake-up calls'.[xx] Let's have a look at why that may be.

Very often women notice changes to their period and menstrual cycle during their forties; shorter, longer, heavier, lighter, more pain, less pain, more exhaustion or bigger mood swings. And for other women it can all seem steady as she goes until periods stop short at menopause. In keeping with the whole menstrual project what is clear is that there is incredible variety in women's experiences.

Very often knowing if you are in peri-menopause is based simply on your age and symptoms. A doctor can take blood tests to check hormone levels to see if peri-menopause is indicated, but commonly the signs are self-assessed.

There are two fundamental stages in the transition of peri-menopause:

- **The Early Stage** can begin in some women in their thirties but most often it starts around age forty to forty-four. This is marked by changes in menstrual flow (more or less) and in the length (shorter, longer, both) of the cycle.

- **The Late Stage** usually occurs when women are in their late forties or early fifties when they begin to experience missed or erratic periods, until they finally stop completely.

For many women peri-menopause is a completely normal gradual process and not particularly symptomatic. While for many others hot flushes and night sweats, insomnia, fatigue and loss of zest, anxiety, mood swings, irritability and depression, decreased libido, vaginal dryness, breast tenderness, bloating and increased PMS symptoms litter their days and nights.

> *Since peri-menopause began I wish I wouldn't bleed so much: on clothes, on bed linen, on the carpet, on furniture. I have to take a towel with me to the movies to sit on so I don't have an 'accident'. I wish I knew more about my body and what's going on. I wish I didn't dread it. I don't ever want to go to a hospital ever again. I want to go back to zero pills-no painkillers, no iron tablets, no mefenamic acid. Ever.*

The hormonal heat haze

Hot flushes are still not fully understood, and researchers have only recently determined that measured hormonal changes take place during a flush. During late stage peri-menopause and menopause diminished oestrogen causes an increase in the levels of the hormones FSH and LH. The brain centre that secretes these hormones, the hypothalamus, directs many bodily functions, including body temperature, sleep patterns, metabolic rate, mood and reaction to stress, so with higher levels of FSH and LH all these can be disturbed, including causing the common 'hot flush'.

Other hormones and biochemical levels also fluctuate in response to altered oestrogen levels. As we know, hormones don't operate in a vacuum and a rise or fall in any one creates a cascading interplay that can affect multiple bodily functions.

For most women if they experience symptoms and discomforts associated with peri-menopause these can be managed well through lifestyle changes. These may be reviewing good diet and nutrition principles, thoughtful and enjoyable exercise and prioritising time for relaxation and creativity. That said around ten per cent of women experience particularly difficult peri-menopausal symptoms requiring expert health professional assessment and support.

For many women peri-menopause also provides an opportunity to take stock and make lifestyle changes that will improve their wellbeing in preparation for the next phase of life. How a woman navigates these changes, how she gives meaning to these processes, how she practises awareness of them and engages with gentle self-care will all impact how this phase is for her.

Menopause is considered *early* if it occurs under the age of forty-five. *Premature* menopause happens when periods stop in a woman under forty and can include girls as young as sixteen. That said, premature menopause is the experience of only one per cent of the female population.

Women who have a family history of premature menopause may be genetically more susceptible to starting the wind-down early.

Premature menopause can also be a result of surgical removal of the ovaries. While a hysterectomy does not necessarily cause menopause, a hysterectomy that involves removal of both ovaries (a bilateral oophorectomy) does cause immediate menopause – no ovaries, no more cyclical hormonal cascade to trigger egg maturation and ovulation.

Some types of cancer radiation and chemotherapy treatments can also induce menopause as can medical conditions such as certain autoimmune disorders, like rheumatoid arthritis and Graves disease. Genetic disorders such as Turner syndrome that cause ovarian abnormalities can also predispose a woman to early or premature menopause.

An end and a new beginning

Unless a woman's ovaries are damaged by certain diseases or cancer treatments, or if they're surgically removed, menopause is a completely natural process, just as menarche is, and a normal part of aging.

THE BIOLOGICAL INTEGRITY OF MENSTRUATION

In most cases, after years of a menstrual cycle, and perhaps a few years of erratic periods, it all stops. No more cycling hormones. No more pads, cramps, leaks, tampons or PMS, no more contraception. This permanent pause may be greeted with joy or grief or a shrug, or many shades in between and often several at once. *Whatever the case, what now?*

For some women menopause heralds a heavy load of life-disturbing emotional and physical symptoms, for others just a few of these, and some may simply notice a few mild challenges alongside welcome changes. The latter can include relief from pain and heavy blood loss, refreshed energy levels, greater mental clarity and emotional steadiness. Renewal.

Physiologically and biochemically there are significant changes that come with the cessation of periods. While our bodies don't cease to produce sex hormones the levels and proportions do alter.

What we do know is this: oestrogen and progesterone levels decline significantly as they are no longer produced by the ovaries as part of the hormonal cascade of the menstrual cycle. That said some will continue to be made by the adrenal glands, fat cells, skin, and brain, but nowhere near the levels of the cycling years.

Testosterone is still produced by the ovaries after menopause and in the same quantities as before, for a few years at least. While testosterone is not as major a hormonal player as oestrogen and progesterone were during the cycling years, as these are markedly reduced after menopause and testosterone remains the same, the proportions of these sex hormones to each other is significantly reset.

Is it thanks to relatively higher testosterone to oestrogen that many women speak of post-menopausal life as characterised by assertiveness, clarity of purpose and being less swayed by the wants and needs of others? Could this be the hormonal precursor of the no-nonsense postmenopausal woman? It certainly can be blamed for an increase in facial whiskers!

When a woman reaches menopause, she will have spent a total of *six and a half to seven years* menstruating, shed approximately a half to one litre of menstrual blood for every cycling year, and bought and used seventeen shopping trolleys of pads and tampons, more or less. Innovations in usable menstrual products like cups, period underwear and cloth pads may significantly change this latter image in years to come.

Menopause is official when a woman has experienced a full twelve months without a period, marking the end of menstruation and fertility. Technically menopause refers to the permanent 'pause' immediately after the last period. The word comes from the Greek 'mens' for month and 'pausis' for cessation. Simply the end of periods.

> *I was very fortunate to be on sabbatical while going through menopause – I think the transitioning actually enhanced the work I was doing at the time; fortunately, I was able to set my own schedule. It helped to be able to sleep in if I'd been awake during the night; and I was able to cry as much or as often as it came up.*

However, as there is a considerable delay to knowing when this 'pause' occurred, and perhaps after several false calls, this contributes to the nebulousness surrounding menopause, so the term has come to be understood as the whole symptomatic time after periods stop. Though the term postmenopausal more accurately refers to the time after which a woman no longer experiences any symptoms of the menopausal change.

As women can now expect to live significantly more post-menopausal years than ever before more thoughtful consideration and research is necessary to better understand what it means to live well during these years. In Australia women reach menopause at around 50, with 90 per cent having arrived there by 55. As women now have a life expectancy of more than 80 we can expect to be alive for some 30 or more years in a postmenopausal state. How do we want to frame that and how do we best live it?

The signs and symptoms of menopause

The biochemical markers that cause the signs and symptoms of menopause include the following:

- An increase in FSH and decreases in oestradiol and inhibin are the major endocrine changes that occur during the transition to menopause.

- While FSH is the diagnostic marker for ovarian cessation both FSH and LH rise to higher levels than those seen in the surge during the menstrual cycle.

- Fluctuation in levels of hormones is very small now and the quantity is also considerably lower than during the menstruating years.

- Gonadotropin (GnRH) secretion increases dramatically after menopause.

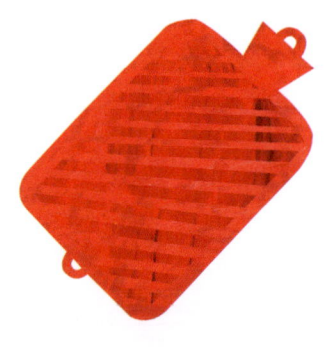

The most prominent symptoms of menopause include:

- *Hot flushes and night sweats*, which may be felt as an intense build-up in body heat, followed by sweating and chills. Some women report accompanying anxiety as the sensation builds. In most cases, hot flushes will occur for three to five years, although for some women they linger for years after menopause. Women who have surgical removal of both ovaries, may have more severe hot flushes than women who enter menopause naturally.

- *Insomnia* may be caused by hot flushes/night sweats or be indicative of general hormonal fluctuations.

- *Mood swings, depression and irritability* may occur due to hormonal changes and many women certainly find the transition to menopause psychologically stressful. However, once a woman has reached menopause depression and mood swings are no more common than before, and many women who have experienced psychological effects of PMS may experience significant improvement.

The most common signs of menopause:

- *Thinning, drying and reduced elasticity of the vaginal walls* may result from the decrease in oestrogen. The vagina becomes shorter, narrower and lubricates less easily, all of which can in turn cause pain during penetrative sex.

- *The uterus shrinks* to the size of a small pear as it us no longer plumped up by oestrogen and progesterone and their cyclic fluctuations.

- *The ovary diminishes* in size and is no longer palpable during a gynaecologic examination.

- *Labia can lose their fatty tissue* and become smaller.

- *Endometriosis and adenomyosis are alleviated* because monthly hormones are no longer triggering them.

- *Numerous changes of puberty now reverse* causing thinning of pubic hair, lightening of nipple colour and thickening of the waist.

So, what does this mean? We know that hormones can have different functions at different times, and we know that the study of hormones, endocrinology, is still in its infancy, as has been noted by endocrinologists. With this in mind it is difficult to imagine that the surge in FSH and LH in menopause and beyond is only due to the pituitary trying to kick-start the ovaries, *for decades after the ovaries have shut up shop!* What we can say is that the hormonal profile of women after

> We need to completely re-think menopause. My son, who is a nurse, said with resignation, "Let's face it Mum, when you reach menopause, it's game over…"! NOT SO!!! **It doesn't mean that we become dried up asexual has-beens!** That we will no longer be valid or attractive or even useful! If we interpret it as distressing, depressing, disabling and debilitating, it will be all of those things and worse. It isn't easy, that's for sure. We need to fight it every step of the way.

menopause is most certainly much different to before. We do need to understand much much more about what this profile means in positive terms, not just as lack or loss or dysfunction.

We know that hormones have physical as well as emotional impacts, and that by triggering an event at a particular site the hormones released can impact our whole being. We know that hormones are incredibly powerful in infinitesimally small quantities – some as low as one millionth of a microgram (one picogram) per mL – and all are measured in parts per million, billion or trillion. So, during this time of change as hormones fluctuate these can be felt strongly as a hot flush, a night sweat or a wave of anxiety or disorientation.

Menopause: disease and deficiency?

The pathologising of menopause and the post-menopausal woman has been a multi-pronged assault, none more clearly defined than by Dr John Studd, consultant gynaecologist at King's College Hospital, London, who, when visiting New Zealand in 1987 as a guest speaker at a gynaecology conference, called menopause 'a multi-system deficiency disorder' which affects the skin, skeleton, pelvis, bladder, heart and brain. He called menopausal women 'these wretched women' undergoing 'general atrophy'. [xxi]

This definition of menopause by Studd and others has in many ways become the dominant narrative and it is easy to see the colossal commercial potential in doing so. A simple internet search for information on menopause almost exclusively throws up stories of depletion, failure, loss, symptoms to treat and the drugs to treat them with. While of course there may be symptoms and many women do have a sense of loss, this narrative alone is woefully inadequate given that this change heralds a brand new phase of life with opportunities as well as challenges, no less important and rich than any other.

In fact, there may be at least as many different stories of what menopause means as there are cultures. Rajput women of India at menopause emerge from *purdah* (the seclusion and veiling of women) and are free to socialise, visit other households and drink with men if they so choose. Lugbara women in Uganda become a 'big woman' and are given considerable authority among their kin. In Māori society, older women become a *kuia*, a person of veneration and respect. Curiously women in these societies, at least traditionally, reported few, if any, troubling symptoms of menopause.

The nature of the end of fertility

While the postmenopausal ovary has shrunk and no longer produces eggs, it represents years of life and experience and a metaphorical rich kernel of nourishing wisdom.

At her first bleeding a woman meets her power.

During her bleeding years she practices it.

At menopause she becomes it.

— American First Nations saying [xxii]

By menopause our ovaries are covered with tiny white scars, one for each ovulation so, were we to follow this American First Nations principle, we could perhaps count the incremental wisdom gained through our ovulating years by each tiny scar.

To explore menopause further let's also consider: *how common is menopause in the natural world?*

The simple answer is not very, but a longer answer is worth a little detour.

There are some species that have a menstrual cycle in which females live on for a few years after menopause, like lions and baboons, but these former mothers care mostly for their own last offspring, helping to ensure their survival. There are only three species in which females cease having a fertility cycle and who go on living for a long time: humans, elephants, and pilot whales. [xxiii]

Elephants and pilot whales breed to age 40 or so, then live on among their daughters and granddaughters, until around 60 for pilot whales and even older for elephants. In terms of evolutionary biology these older females are known as 'alloparents', because they are bonded to young relatives and are highly sensitive to their signals of need.

Sarah Blaffer Hrdy, a leading sociobiologist who wrote *Mother Nature – Natural Selection and the Female of the Species*, reports that, 'In many species females become increasingly altruistic as they decline in reproductive value. Langur monkeys provide a particularly vivid primate example of old females who become simultaneously more self-sacrificing and more heroic as they age.' [xxiv]

Blaffer Hrdy notes that traditionally where women remain among their kin they also tend to become more altruistic with age. Based on data from peoples like the Hazda and !Kung, older women appear to work harder and more effectively by bringing more gathered food back to camp than they themselves will consume. This economic contribution translates to more reverence for older women in gathering societies, although notably less so in those more focused on hunting or herding where these roles are more commonly performed by men.[xxv]

The figure of the crone was once revered and is now more commonly one of derision. What's this about?

Menopause: the end of the line?

We have a clear need to distinguish menopause from aging and re-position menopause as an event of mid-life, but by no means the only one. While both men and women age, with women there is a tendency to attribute the troublesome aspects of aging with menopause so that menopause tends to be blamed for any difficult aspects of midlife.

Menopause also draws a sharp line that signals the finish of fertility, a line that does not exist for men, at least not in so clearly defined a way. This has a greater impact in a society where a woman's fecundity and youthfulness define her worth. We'll revisit this theme for closer examination later.

Because of the symptomatic and cultural loading of menopause it is especially important to be clear as to what symptoms are caused by peri-menopausal and menopausal hormonal changes, what symptoms belong to other causes (anaemia, thyroid issues, jaundice, high or low blood pressure and diabetes for instance) and what misinformation needs to be stripped away for a woman to understand her changes, her needs and herself. The catch-all approach, where a plethora of health issues are randomly and erroneously attributed to menopause, causes confusion, erodes positive health outcomes and encourages an unnecessarily pessimistic view of menopause. It is clearly not helpful to consider menopause a deficiency disease or a time trial or a sign of diminished capacity. It is a natural, normal event, which also has observable changes attached to it and a wide array of individual experiences, many of which do require specific understanding and support for women to be able to traverse these changes positively. Men also undergo significant hormonal changes during andropause, though generally with less social judgement attached.

We need to completely re-think menopause. My son, who is a nurse, said with resignation, "Let's face it Mum, when you reach menopause, it's game over..."! NOT SO!!! It does not mean that we become dried up asexual has-beens! That we will no longer be valid or attractive or even useful! If we interpret it as distressing, depressing, disabling and debilitating, it will be all of those things and worse. It isn't easy, that's for sure. We need to fight it every step of the way.

As essential as the ovulation-menstruation cycle is for our existence, menopause has also evolved to best ensure the continuation of families and the species. In the modern world this does not always play out as evolution intended, however the specific qualities of the post-fertility, post-menstrual cycling experience for many women affords them the time, energy and attention to make a profound contribution to society and the world on many and varied levels. Women are inherently valuable and important at every stage of their lives, and what we know of the menstrual and post-menstrual life cycle reflects this.

No body is an island

At the beginning of this section we wanted to create a plain-speak treatment of our bodies at work and we hope that it has worked, for you. We don't expect you to memorise every last detail, and there won't be a pop quiz! However, if there is anything we can all take away from this, it is surely that menstruation has its own internal deep complexity and inherent value. Hopefully you have the strong impression that the physiological underpinnings of menarche, menstruation and menopause are not in and of themselves inviting revulsion and opprobrium. These processes have a profound integrity. They are intricate, robust, and absolutely essential.

So, what is going on? Why do so many societies still treat menstruation and menopause in the negative? How has disgust and revulsion overridden awe and respect? Why has silence and shame been projected onto these most vital functions? The answer lies in understanding the menstrual taboo.

As we've demonstrated, it's vitally important to know what is happening inside our bodies but what about outside of them? We are social beings and we live in communities where our ideas, values and attitudes are shaped collectively to a significant extent. Individual women and girls are subject to many of the same cultural narratives that construct menstruation as inherently shameful or disgusting. This is the menstrual taboo at work. It operates on the whole of society, not just on the individual.

THE BIOLOGICAL INTEGRITY OF MENSTRUATION

As we'll discuss in the next section, taboos are powerful drivers of social values. They create invisible boundaries and help to instruct people how to behave in a society, outside of their own ideas and even those of their immediate family. The menstrual taboo shapes and defines our collective attitudes towards menstruation, resulting in a pervasive culture of menstrual shame. In order to revolutionise menstrual culture, we need to shake it up, tackle it head on. First, we need to see it. Then we can name it, strip it of its power and finally dismantle it for good.

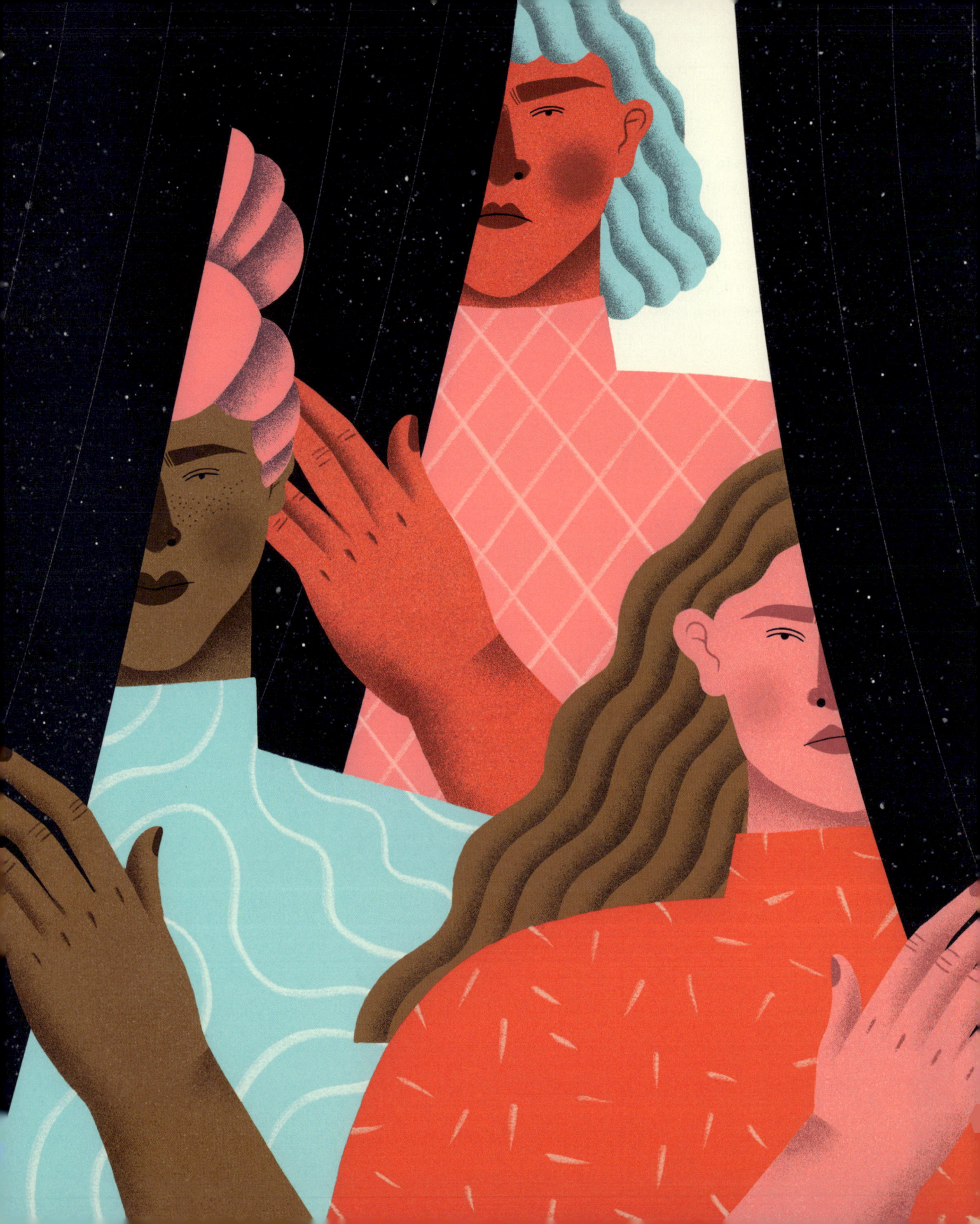

A PERVASIVE MENSTRUAL TABOO

WOMEN ARE RELIABLE NARRATORS OF THEIR OWN LIVES. We believe them when they tell us that their experience of menstruation and menopause has often been difficult, confusing, painful, embarrassing, and generally negative. We believe them when they say it is hard to talk about menstruation. But we don't accept it has to be this way, because we can also see the menstrual cycle for what it is: an important biological process of the body that not only has the potential to create life but is a decisive indicator of overall physical health. Women and girls are trapped inside a deep paradox: the very thing that guarantees all human life is something they are asked to condemn as humiliating and disgusting.

> *I still avoid staying at friend's places if I have my period. I don't mind discussing 'the period' topic but I definitely don't like colleagues or friends knowing that I have my period. I also prefer that other people keep that information to themselves.*

> *Even now I don't tell anyone other than hubby or doctor when I have my period – I feel so secretive about it, perhaps I still have some shame or embarrassment. I hide tampons when I need to go to the bathroom rather than just grab them out of my handbag. I feel that my teenage life especially would've been easier if there was no stigma or silence around the topic of menstruation.*

> *I feel like no one wants to hear about periods and like it's somehow a separate thing from day to day life. We hide it all from such a young age, learn to think we are dirty and need to stay clean, learn that no one wants to hear about our pain or fears. We've done such a poor job of that for ourselves.*

There are two realities here that are equally valid. The inescapable biological truth is that our entire existence depends on the menstrual cycle. Quite literally it is a powerful and positive life force. The other undeniable fact is the difficulty many women have in dealing with it.

It seems to occupy a curious place in our collective psyche. Instead of awe for the life-giving properties of the menstrual cycle, our culture demeans it, fostering and perpetuating feelings of visceral disgust, revulsion and distrust, along with inconvenience, boredom and resentment. Cultural practice shrouds menstruation in negativity, and increasingly it is framed as a process with little or dubious value. We are discouraged from talking about it or seeing it as meaningful. Instead of respect and reverence, we are raised to feel embarrassed and awkward about menstruation, whether we menstruate or not.

There is such massive incongruity between these two realities, but the latter is not less real just because it is subjective and variable. We can see clearly that there is a problem, and that these attitudes result in girls and women feeling ashamed and humiliated.

Of all the powerful and even majestic things our bodies do it is bewildering that the menstrual cycle is so stigmatised and misunderstood; shrouded in secrecy, and subject to prohibitive cultural rules and practices which cloak menstruation in taboo.

The idea of a taboo

It helps us at this stage to focus first and in general terms on the concept of a taboo. It's interesting that the word itself only entered our lexicon relatively recently, even though societies throughout history have nonetheless enacted and enforced various prohibitions on particular ideas and cultural practices. What are they and why do we have them?

'Taboo' entered the English language after Captain James Cook's time in Tonga in 1777, when he encountered the concept of tapu, a complex system of reverence and reproach in Tongan culture, involving negotiation of what is sacred, untouchable and sacrosanct. Many cultures have similar ideas and systems, and religious concepts like kadesh and haram are some of the means by which taboos are taught and policed, in Judaism and Islam, for example. Through the cultural education of prohibition and punishment, a taboo will be rigorously taught and adhered to within a culture, and by adulthood, every person in that culture will be aware of its importance and power.

A taboo will live or die by the number of people who obey it, and its strength and resilience depends on its popular understanding and broad social agreement.[i]

There are punishments for breaking them, and personal costs in keeping them. It is this weighing of the personal losses or gains against the society's expectations and demands that give taboos their cultural logic. Importantly, taboos are taught to upcoming generations as they grow up, so they absorb their import at an impressionable time, when the taboo also represents the cultural cachet of adulthood. Children become willing participants in the maintenance, who grow up to be effective gatekeepers of the taboo, without necessarily re-examining it from an adult perspective.

It is useful to think about how taboos are built up, and how they are broken down. There have been taboos in our culture that have lost their potency and relevance as more people broke them and fewer people considered them worth upholding. People have questioned whether a taboo should exist, in some cases have broken it, and social change has followed. A short list of examples might include: women showing their ankles, married women and mothers in the paid workforce, breastfeeding in public, people of the same gender showing physical affection in a romantic sense, men hugging each other (in a romantic or platonic sense), men crying in front of others for a

> Even now I don't tell anyone other than hubby or doctor when I have my period – I feel so secretive about it, perhaps I still have some shame or embarrassment. I hide tampons when I need to go to the bathroom rather than just grab them out of my handbag. I feel that my teenage life especially would've been easier if there was no stigma or silence around the topic of menstruation.

reason other than death or war or sport. Progress towards change can be sporadic and intermittent but we can see the pattern at work – a taboo builds up over time and becomes difficult to question, no matter how illogical and incompatible with contemporary beliefs. It is questioned, challenged, broken and eventually consigned to history. This is the life cycle of a taboo.

We should add that a taboo in itself is not necessarily allied to a cause of moral purity. Taboos are not intrinsically 'bad' things. Like all social constructs invented by humans in organizing themselves, like road rules or democracy or calendars, they can be very useful and important. For instance, in Māori society elders called *tohunga* used *tapu* to prevent the overuse of environmental resources, by declaring a reef off limits for fishing. In most cultures, incest and paedophilia are taboo, which has origins in evolutionary survival but now involves a strong moral dimension as reflected in cultural attitudes and laws. We can see the soundness and merit in these taboos, and many other taboos around food consumption, for example, also have their roots in preventing contamination and ensuring the survival of the group.

While it's true that some taboos should be upheld, it helps us to remember that they aren't necessarily maintained because people consider them deeply or revise their views on the subject often. It's entirely conceivable that a taboo remains in place precisely because the cultural norms they produce seem inevitable, unchanging and unquestionable.

Taboos are often separate from laws and may not be enforced in the same way. This means they can be codified into behaviours and actions through the power of cultural norms. Cultural norms are the customs and practices within a social group, often understood as unwritten rules that we learn to follow from childhood into adult life. These norms might adapt and change from one generation to the next, although some are more resilient and inflexible. They may also change from place to place, with travellers finding that what is acceptable and welcome in one country may be unacceptable and frowned upon in another. You might learn not to wear shoes inside a Japanese home, for example, or to tip American wait staff a certain percentage of the whole bill. Cultural norms are learned, observed and passed on, often absorbed without ever being questioned, examined or considered deeply.

Everyone around me was always a bit ashamed to talk about it, like it was something embarrassing. I had terribly painful heavy periods and about five years ago was diagnosed with endometriosis, but no GP had ever talked to me about that being a possibility. I can talk to my male partner and mother about period issues but can't even talk to my sister or female friends about it much because they're so embarrassed. I have always found periods to be a negative experience, as well as inconvenient and even disempowering because of the stupid social stigma about it. I still feel uncomfortable buying sanitary products at the supermarket because I don't want others to know I'm menstruating. I know this is ridiculous, but I just have so much shame about periods.

The menstrual taboo has produced all kinds of unwritten rules and they commonly go unexamined and unnoticed, until they are challenged or broken. Girls and women are taught, often by other women and girls, through cultural absorption or by committing a social faux pas, that speaking in open and honest terms about your period is unwelcome in most interpersonal interactions, even when necessary. They will often use euphemisms to talk about it ('women's troubles') or opt instead for a face-saving lie (stomach ache), or even just 'soldier on', when it might be more logical to simply say, 'I have my period'. They may automatically abstain from sex while they menstruate, accepting the cultural norm that period blood is anathema to physical intimacy and sexual activity.

Another cultural norm around menstruation is the assumption that all menstrual products are disposable; tampons, pads, and panty liners are what most Australian women use to manage their periods. The taboo limits conversation and therefore works against a wider awareness of more economical, reusable and sustainable options. It is interesting to consider that in North America tampons most often come with telescopic applicators, meaning that the tampon can be inserted without the woman touching her genitals. While we know that cultural norms around menstruation do vary from culture to culture, the menstrual taboo cuts across almost every society, language and country. This is an indication of its immense power.

The menstrual taboo across time and culture

But menstruation is not automatically shrouded in taboo in all cultures everywhere. The good news is that there are some societies and communities, past and present, where it is instead recognised as a positive life force; the font of life; and something to be honoured and revered. There are cultures that value menstruation as sacred, holy, and speaking to the power of creation, even practicing holistic and thoughtful celebration of menstruation, especially menarche and menopause. In Assam, India, pilgrims to the Kamakhya temple can see the titular deity known as The Bleeding Goddess being worshipped to honour the shakti power (in this case, of the womb) in every woman. Ulithi women of the Pacific retire to an *ipul* (women's house), but despite being technically sequestered, use the time to socialise and enjoy a rest from their usual labours, with the *ipul* itself becoming a de facto community centre for women in the village.

But there are societies and places where the opposite applies, including our own, where the menstrual taboo is real, powerful and pervasive. To grapple with it and see how deeply it can be ingrained in a cultural context, we need to consider the origins and logic of the taboo, as well as what makes it so widespread and resilient. Where does it come from? What does it mean? Who upholds it? And how does the menstrual taboo have a deleterious effect on our whole society, but especially on women and girls?

We can trace the menstrual taboo back in time, through the history of ancient civilisations and the development of organised religion. Religious tradition and observance also play an important part in forming social and cultural norms regarding menarche, menstruation and menopause, and examining these can really help us understand how the taboo functions to shut down, challenge or critique.

Anti-menstrual sentiment can be found in the key texts of all the major faiths: Christianity, Islam, Judaism and Hinduism have all preached that menstrual blood, and women who menstruate, are unclean, impure, and are responsible for everything from failing crops to contaminated meat. Of course, most religious texts are complex in meaning and scholars spend decades unpacking and re-translating single sentences or even words, but the prohibitions and limitations placed on menstruating women are clear. Given how much of the world's population adheres to one or other of these religions, the effect of these prohibitions is felt widely and deeply. Institutions and indeed whole nations are founded on theocratic principles, to a greater or lesser extent, and even a largely secular country like Australia carries the vestiges of a Judeo-Christian tradition in its laws, customs and culture.

The first five books of the Christian Bible, Genesis, Exodus, Leviticus, Deuteronomy and Numbers, form the Pentateuch, which is also known as the Torah in Judaism. Leviticus 15: 19-33 describes menstruation and women, stating that 'if a woman have an issue, and her issue in her flesh be blood, she shall be put apart seven days: and whosoever toucheth her shall be unclean … ', and describes the menstruating woman as a figure to be feared and reviled, including a prohibition on her clothing, food, and anything else she touches.

Orthodox Jewish women acquire the status of *niddah* when they menstruate, meaning literally to move away or separate, but also translated as 'uncleanness' and related to the concept of ritual impurity. She may not touch or be touched by her husband for seven days, at which time she'll undergo a *mikveh*, the ritual bath to cleanse and purify her from the pollution. A Jewish girl is sometimes slapped across the face at menarche, by her mother, who was slapped across the face by hers, as a way of marking the occasion. The meaning of this tradition is not agreed on, with interpretations varying from the slap scaring off evil spirits, to the idea that it brought blood to the cheeks to boost circulation!

When a practicing Muslim woman gets her period, she may recite a *Kalima*, an article of faith, to begin her ban from fasting, reciting daily prayers or touching the Holy Qur'an. Menstruating women may be prevented from entering mosques and joining the *Hajj*. Hindu women are also considered dangerous and unclean when they menstruate, and are barred from entering many temples, or touching certain food and drink.

But it isn't just religion that has constructed the menstruating woman as soiled, inferior and dangerous. We can also see the taboo in action throughout the broader sweep of history – there are long traditions in many cultures of vilifying or diminishing menstruation and the bleeding woman, as part of a general fear of female sexuality, reproductive power and the bodies that were capable of such 'mystery'.

The Greek philosopher Aristotle (380-322 BCE) expounded a theory of women as incomplete males; 'as it were, a deformity', and regarded menstrual blood as a lesser form of semen. The Roman Pliny the Elder wrote *Natural History* several hundred years later in 77-79 CE, claiming that contact with menstrual blood 'turns new wine sour, crops touched by it become barren, grafts die, seed in gardens are dried up, the fruit of trees fall off, the edge of steel and the gleam of ivory are dulled, hives of bees die, even bronze and iron are at once seized by rust, and a horrible smell fills the air; to taste it drives dogs mad and infects their bites with an incurable poison'.[ii] Tertullian, the 2nd century Christian scholar who has been called the 'founder of Western theology', wrote 'Woman is a temple built over a sewer'.

A menstrual taboo today?

So why is menstrual blood so mortifying to so many people? Why do those menstruating try to hide the fact from others? Why do many women feel disconnected and demeaned by the process? And why do people see it and react in a way so disproportionate to the reality? Are there power politics at work here? What does the distant past have to do with how we view menstruation, and menstruating women, now? If we have evolved beyond the archaic notions of people who didn't know any better, why are we still disgusted by menses? And why is this discrimination so ingrained and deeply held?

> *I still feel ashamed about periods and I don't understand why.*

> *In a way, it feels to me like so many women are survivors of a 'great cataclysm' of sorts. The wound, collectively, feels that extreme.*

The ambiguity and incongruity at work here ultimately stems from a fundamental belief system and its values, which underpin the patriarchal organisation of our society. Culturally and politically, our society has relied heavily on traditional ideas of what roles men and women should perform. Whether we call it sexism, patriarchy, or 'just the way things are', for most of human history, men have found their power in society commensurate with their ability to be dominant, commanding and controlling (often physically), while women have been largely prescribed roles of wives and mothers, and valued for their mildness, compassion and nurturance (in spite of their physical 'weakness' they have been recognised as contributing meaningfully, but only in very specific ways). Men have been trusted and encouraged to wield authority and influence across society, as leaders, legislators, industrialists and other economic drivers. Women are 'the other', seen as inferior, 'the gentler sex', assigned lesser roles; all the time negotiating their needs (such as reproductive rights) from a position of less power. In such a patriarchal world, women's bodies are the locus of huge anxiety and contestation, because they are simultaneously desired, feared, hated, scrutinised, coveted and revered for their many powers – there is envy and resentment of a body that can create and sustain life, be a source of longing and ecstasy, and has an internal cycle connected to the seasons, the cosmos and everything that grows. Women's bodies *are* incredible, which is why many cultures worshipped them, but it's this intense power that also drives a patriarchal impulse to control them.

To criticise patriarchal organisation is not to condemn men, but rather to point out the complex, subterranean and largely invisible structures in place that distribute power from one group to the other, through an interdependent set of cultural mechanisms. The menstrual taboo is one of those devices. It reifies male strength and power at the same time as holding women back by making them anxious about their bodies and causing them to struggle with bodily confidence from the time they begin menstruating. It reinforces the false idea that men are somehow superior, rational and capable while suggesting women are inherently unstable, emotional and less rational. And it stops women from seeing the injustice of this treatment and from agitating for change, by layering silence and secrecy over the suffering.

> *My mother was very prudish and uptight about any bodily function. I was given a book and told to go away and read it. My father and brother gave me little privacy and were mocking about it, quite shaming. I learnt to be very secretive and never went to them if I needed any help – I always bought my own products.*

> *My mother had a highly negative perspective about being a woman. She wanted me to be a boy. She hated menstruation and said women are damned to bleed 'like pigs'. I was really angry but didn't know why. Now I think it's because I felt rejected and somehow hated along with my menstruating body.*

> *'Women's stuff' was not discussed openly in my family even between women, and if it was absolutely necessary then semi-encrypted messages were whispered far away from men's ears. Being a Catholic family there was heavy programming about sexuality and that genitals were disgusting. It was also quite a patriarchal household where the feminine was not valued. So, I learnt that anything to do with my vagina was a source of shame, anxiety and embarrassment.*

> *My mother was sexually abused, and her shame and awkwardness were part of my upbringing. Sexuality and femininity were always shrouded with shame and embarrassment, and I've been unpacking this forever it seems.*

Patriarchal systems not only create an environment in which the menstrual taboo thrives, but they reinforce and strengthen it; and everyone plays a role, including other women and girls who are more likely to pass on their internalised shame, to become a tormentor, to judge the way people manage their periods, to project their feelings about menstruation onto other's experience of it. Mothers, sisters, grandmothers, aunts, neighbours, teachers, classmates, nurses, babysitters, early learning educators, colleagues, managers and strangers in the public toilet – they all have the power to either reproduce or reinforce the menstrual taboo. Men have this power too. Everyone, however, has the capacity and the choice to challenge and work against the taboo.

The menstrual taboo in action: pervasive, (ever)present and harmful

The menstrual taboo cannot be reduced to a single practice; it is a complex social phenomenon, manifesting in a network of overlapping and intersecting discriminations and penalties: financial, social, cultural, sexual, physical, professional, and economic; some subtle and invisible, others direct and obvious. Where does the taboo operate? Put simply, everywhere.

Through the enforcement of social sanctions and cultural norms, girls take social cues from a young age that their period is something secret, shameful and stigmatised, and women carry this message with them throughout their lives. There aren't many parts of a girl's or woman's life that aren't affected by it, and indeed boys and men suffer its ill effects too. Pervasive does not mean that everybody experiences it equally, but that it presents everywhere in observable, definable and significant ways. When we look at the lives of girls and women, listening to what they told us, we

> My mother was very prudish and uptight about any bodily function. I was given a book and told to go away and read it. My father and brother gave me little privacy and were mocking about it, quite shaming. **I learnt to be very secretive** and never went to them if I needed any help – I always bought my own products.

can see distinct clear realms; all facets of a woman's life are adversely affected and made more difficult because of how this taboo functions.

So how do we begin to unpack this? When we look at the different spheres that girls and women inhabit, something troubling unfolds – the menstrual taboo frames menstruation in such negative terms, that girls have little choice but to absorb these cultural messages, which they can then carry for an entire lifetime, resulting in a belief that their menstrual cycle is something to resent, mistrust, and even be ashamed of.

Whether she is at home with her family, at school with her peers and trusted carers, in romantic relationships, at her workplaces, working out her household budget, seeing a doctor, or making consumer decisions, the menstrual taboo is making her life more difficult, whether she registers this or not. The combined effect of the taboo's ever-present and pervasive nature ensures an oppressive silence. The taboo can drive a wedge between a woman and her body, creating negativity and conflict within her sense of self. While many women have worked towards a place of period positivity, the taboo still has the capacity to inhibit and harm. It can place limits on her, or interfere with her personal relationships, placing obstacles in the way of genuine intimacy and mutual respect.

Hiding the truth of her menstruation from teachers, employers, partners, colleagues and even friends consumes significant mental and emotional energy, even contributing to anxiety and exhaustion. She will often find that medical care lacks responsiveness and won't help her move towards a true understanding of her cycle and its connection to her overall health. She may encounter the taboo in the supermarket aisle, as a financial penalty exacted on her each time she buys essential supplies (often deemed by regulators to be non-essential luxury items attracting an extra tax, as was the case in Australia until recently). These already expensive items are purchased repeatedly, throughout her life, to manage this normal, natural and blameless function of her body.

She could meet it in her bedroom; if her period arrives during sex, the taboo might cause a rupture in the connection and trust so necessary for everybody involved to feel safe and respected. She suffers under the taboo again if she struggles through a day of commitments while dealing with searing pain and low energy, instead of just telling everyone that she needs to stay home and rest. To appreciate the pervasiveness and impact of the menstrual taboo let's consider all the spheres in which women and girls are affected.

Home ground disadvantage: meeting the taboo

Our research told us that women and girls frequently experienced real alienation and anxiety around their periods, with the attitudes often starting and being reinforced at home. The findings suggest clearly that home is the most likely place for girls to experience menarche, followed by school. So how girls are prepared, long before their first period, and how the event is treated when it arrives, has a lasting impact – for better or worse – on a girl's relationship with her menstrual cycle and her body.

Every time she has a period at home; or talks about it, or asks for help, or requests supplies, is an opportunity for the menstrual taboo to be perpetuated or challenged. Remembering also that there may be a number of menstruators in the house, the culture within that home with regard to menstruation has a profound influence on all children, whether they get periods or not.

> *I was at home alone when my period came for the first time. I cried and thought I may be dying.*

> *Yay I'm a woman. And oh crap.*

> *I wish someone had explained to me that I was having period cramps. I thought that my internal organs were bursting.*

Our research suggests that a large majority of girls learn from their mothers, who bring their own emotional experience to their menstrual education of daughters, and the messages they get can be a mixture of sage advice, value judgments and anxiety. Our respondents shared so many variations on the same negative and sometimes frightening themes, like 'you are a woman now and this signals the beginning of your adult life' and 'you are responsible for "dealing with it" every month so don't tell anyone that you are menstruating or talk about it openly', which you can well imagine might be very confronting for a 10 to 15 year old girl who does not feel prepared. Girls were told 'don't let the blood leak onto your clothes', 'you don't need extra rest, different food, or easier routines' as well as the more explicitly negative conversations along the lines of 'blood is dirty, smelly, embarrassing and wicked'.

Some women also reported having beautiful connections with their mothers about periods, but they were very much in the minority. And the menstrual taboo also meant that while in some instances mum planned celebrations and offered congratulations, girls were still able to read her negativity towards her own period (or the household's) and that undermined the verbal message. Kids pick up on so much more than what we tell them to their face! And here we are talking about girls of anywhere from eight to fifteen years old, an incredibly diverse group but not one especially equipped to decode the difference between mum's anxiety, the world's, and their own.

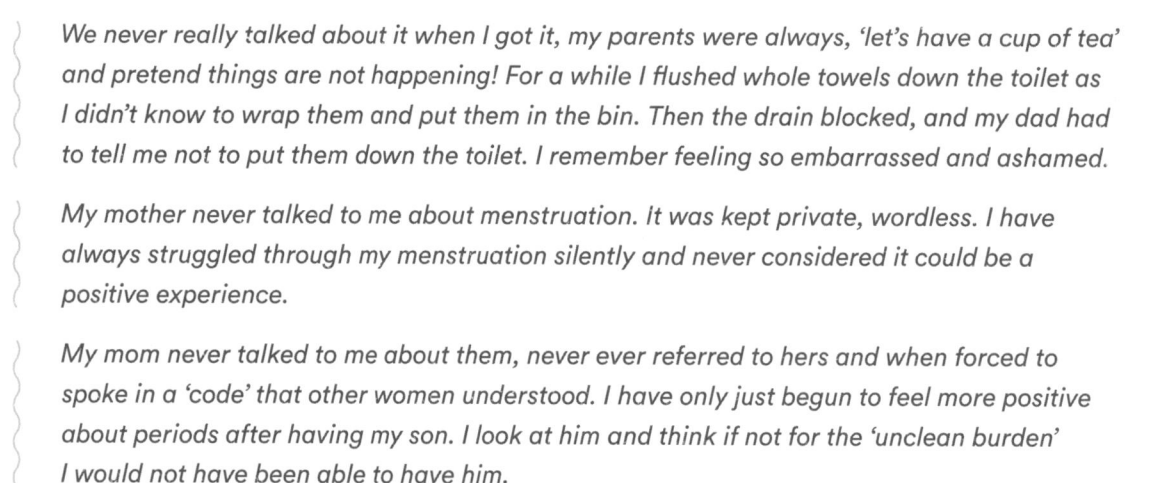

> *We never really talked about it when I got it, my parents were always, 'let's have a cup of tea' and pretend things are not happening! For a while I flushed whole towels down the toilet as I didn't know to wrap them and put them in the bin. Then the drain blocked, and my dad had to tell me not to put them down the toilet. I remember feeling so embarrassed and ashamed.*

> *My mother never talked to me about menstruation. It was kept private, wordless. I have always struggled through my menstruation silently and never considered it could be a positive experience.*

> *My mom never talked to me about them, never ever referred to hers and when forced to spoke in a 'code' that other women understood. I have only just begun to feel more positive about periods after having my son. I look at him and think if not for the 'unclean burden' I would not have been able to have him.*

Far from wanting to 'blame the mother' as so many analyses are wont to do, we are seeking an empathic approach to mothers, by recognising that they, like all of us, carry the marks of the menstrual taboo from their own menarche and menstruating lives, and this hurts them too. That this pain would be transmitted to their daughters is understandable, even with a mother's best effort to support her daughter. She may not even be aware of what is being transferred. The taboo often prevents women from examining their attitudes towards their own menarche and menstruation, so that they may unknowingly pass on their negative residual feelings to their daughters.

But of course, mothers are not the only parents. Our research found that fathers were down the bottom of the list of places a girl might consult to find out information about her period, after mum at number one, followed by school, friends, books, magazines, sister, the internet, other relative, and television. Again, this is not intended to shame or judge fathers, only to observe the reality that they are often separate from their daughter's experience of menstruation. Only brothers scored lower, which might also trouble us (as should the fact that popular culture e.g. television has so little period positivity, considering its influence and reach).

While, of course, many fathers and brothers are empathetic and supportive, large numbers of girls experience the opposite. In one affecting response a woman recalled her realisation, as a girl, that when her dad joked about her mum having PMS or 'angry women who must be on that time of the month', he would now mean her as well. More than one respondent described in painful terms how their physical relationship with their father changed almost immediately after they started getting periods, shifting from an easy familiarity to a standoffish reluctance. Let's just process that: girls of 10 to 15 years of age could feel like they don't get hugs or physical affection from their dad anymore, after they start menstruating.

> *In my traditional ethnic family menarche is celebrated in a vague obscure way, never to be mentioned in polite company again. When a girl menstruates for the first time she is presented to society as a 'woman' and must stop childish behaviour.*

> *My mother told me off if I leaked on the sheets overnight, as if I did it on purpose. This happened reasonably often as I bled a lot. Though strangely, when I think about it now, no one ever helped me work out ways to save the sheets with a towel or something. I still feel quite anxious when I have my period.*

> *My dad was religious and told us that labour and menstruation was God's punishment for Eve's sin in the Garden of Eden. My mom countered this by telling us it was simply nature and how we evolved as humans/animals. This left some cognitive dissonance, but the influence of my mom was much stronger since she was a woman and a health professional.*

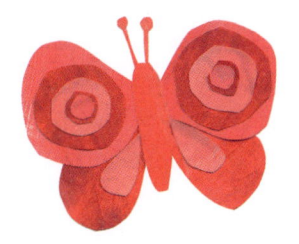

Brothers and even older sisters featured as antagonists to menstruating girls too, with jokes about leakage, smells, weight gain and moodiness being made at home as well as at school. Parents encouraging their daughters to 'get on with it' and 'soldier on' and showing obvious embarrassment and discomfort at conversations about menstruation repeatedly came up in the study. These comments may be intended to promote an atmosphere of capability and resilience, to prevent their daughters being held back by periods, and this makes sense. But it can also contribute to a sense of the invisibility of periods and send the message that the preferred model of the human body is non-menstruating, as more like the male. This may cause girls who would appreciate more comfort and support to squash these needs and feelings without even expressing them. Everything from where products are stored and how they are discussed, to well-meaning 'jokes' and casual comments, can have a strong impact on a child's understanding of what the menstrual cycle means, and pass on the menstrual taboo for life.

School of hard knocks: the stigma intensifies

We spend a lot of our life at school and our data showed that after home it was the next most likely place for girls to experience menarche. After that first period, many more will be navigated around classes, timetables, peer groups and playgrounds. Whether it's the fraught issue of taunting and bullying, access to supplies and amenities, or the attitudes of educators themselves, girls have a lot to deal with during term time. A girl's experience with the menstrual taboo increases within the school environment, and this intensification can have lasting effects on her belief that her period is a source of shame and disgust.

Very few of us had a teacher who modelled comfort and openness when discussing periods. Even fewer went to a school where menstrual education and policy was considered, nuanced, supportive and openly communicated. The data suggest that it is extremely rare. This is certainly as true for the teachers, when they were at school, as it is for the rest of us. The cycle of shame and blame repeats itself, as it does in the home environment. In fact, it's more likely that if menstruation is discussed in classrooms it will reinforce the menstrual taboo rather than deconstruct it, with everything from the obvious discomfort of the educator, through to the possibly uninformed commentary of their peers, contributing to a strong sense of taboo around even the topic itself, let alone the actual process. While they are adept at finding information when it isn't provided, girls still come to understand that talking about menstruation is as unwanted and unwelcome as visible reminders that it exists. If they absorb these attitudes – disrespect, fear, embarrassment, amusement, discomfort and anxiety – and attach them to menstruation, this can become their experience of periods for life.

> *I told the teachers I had my period and suspected other girls did as well, but I was the first one to bring it up. They put a small container in one of the bathrooms on my request, so we could get rid of the tampons. All this happened in a very hush hush way, and I had to tell the other girls about it. Weird.*

Here again we see the menstrual taboo rendering menstruation and the needs of menstruating girls invisible. Where these needs are acknowledged it tends to be a strictly physiological presentation of menstruation as 'what happens when a woman does not conceive', even though a period will be the result of 99.5 per cent of her ovulations for the average woman in a developed country. Sanitary bins may be placed in toilets, but often with no explanation, and in primary schools may not be considered at all. At the time of writing little or no attention is given to the emotional, social and self-care needs of girls approaching, beginning or in the early days of experiencing menstruation, not to mention around half of secondary school populations with ongoing and varied menstrual experiences and needs. Perhaps we expect girls to approach teachers with their needs, and a small number will, but in this instance embarrassment and the menstrual taboo is already well entrenched and most girls will stay silent, uncomfortable, anxious and distracted.

In addition, little or no thought is given to specific menstrual education for boys (again, beyond the strictly biological) and yet this emerged from the data as very important to both girls and women. Boys, after all, share their lives with sisters, mothers, friends and other women, and quite possibly later, men may have girlfriends, wives, daughters and women colleagues. Their positive engagement can make a great difference to girls and women, as well as help boys and men enjoy respectful and happy relationships.

Menstrual education, where it exists, tends toward an inadequate and simplistic 'plumbing' approach, often with deft product placement by industry providers. This leaves girls with little understanding and respect for what their bodies are going through, and for each other. For boys too, the ongoing lack of knowledge leaves them vulnerable to believing schoolyard myths, leading to disrespect and disconnection among their peer group. The results can be devastating for many girls, who not only fear humiliation but also suffer alienation and isolation, on top of the other demands of having a period.

> *If boys got their period it wouldn't be so funny.*

> *I hate that boys act so grossed out even when they see clean tampons. I tell my male friends that I have my period – my girlfriend and I yell it at them because we always seem to get it on the same day.*

> *I'm very jealous of boys. They don't have to go through any of this.*

Girls and women told us repeatedly that school was a scary place to be menstruating, where something like a leak, blood on their clothes, even other students seeing tampons and pads, would result in ruthless teasing, shaming, bullying and harassment of the person menstruating, thus sending the message to all girls that they are just as vulnerable, and they could be next. Our findings were very clear on this difficult reality of the school environment. Of course, girls and women may become excellent supports and confidantes to one another as they grow, but the taboo is still in effect for the many who feel as though they can't connect or empathise around periods. The socialisation of girls at school is complex and variable but the frequency of menstrual shaming among schoolchildren deserves our urgent attention and response.

> *One day in grade school I saw an older girl get a pad from a vending machine. When she realised I was there she threw me up against the bathroom wall and made me swear not to tell anyone that she had her period. Of course, I agreed. I was scared about going to the toilet and scared about periods for a long time after that.*

This can manifest in different ways depending on the social context. A recent report conducted in partnership with the University of Queensland and WaterAid, found that basic menstrual products could be 'unaffordable, unavailable or too shameful to buy for girls and women' in remote Indigenous communities in mainland Australia. There was significant evidence that this was causing girls to miss school during their period, and combined with infrastructural problems like a lack of clean bathrooms, bins and access to running water, we can imagine the extra difficulty experienced by these girls.[iii] Similarly, Essentials 4 Women South Australia established a pilot program to supply schoolgirls with free menstrual products, after it was found that a significant number would simply skip school if they couldn't afford them.[iv] But for all girls of school age, positive menstrual education, modelling comfort and non-judgment about periods, and ensuring access to the supplies they need, would mean serious improvement for their quality of life and educational outcomes.

Beyond our shores, we know that at least 500 million girls and women around the world don't have access to the facilities and products they need to manage their periods, according to a 2015 report from UNICEF and the World Health Organization.[v] UNESCO estimates that one in ten girls in Sub-Saharan Africa miss school during their menstrual cycle.[vi] By some reckonings, this accounts for as much as 20 per cent of a given school year, with many girls dropping out of school altogether once they begin menstruating. In rural India, one in five girls drops out of school after they start menstruating, according to research by Nielsen and Plan India,[vii] and of the 355 million menstruating girls and women in the country, just 12 per cent have access to pads. In the UK, an enquiry into truancy found that 'period poverty' was a major cause of absenteeism among girls who, in many cases, did not want to miss school but had no choice, and we know that the same dire situation faces Australian schoolgirls too.[viii]

So, when we think about girls and women, and who are the major influences, supporters and important figures in their lives – parents, partners, teachers, bosses, doctors, friends, siblings, colleagues – how many of these do girls and women feel comfortable talking to about their periods?

Would girls and women feel safe and welcome to mention their period to all these people? Or ask them important questions about it? Or are we letting girls and women down? That's not people being uncaring or judgmental, that's the menstrual taboo stopping us from having normal, open dialogue about something important that affects all of us. Put it this way, until a schoolchild can ask their school principal for a tampon, with the same nonchalance as if asking for a band-aid or a stapler, then we have work to do.

Connecting despite disconnection: sex and relationships

We know that the way menarche is handled and responded to has a massive impact on every girl, and woman, for the rest of her life. We know that the attitudes that the girl absorbs around her menarche are going to inform her relationship with her body, and the interaction of her body with other bodies, far into her future. When we think about it in that sense, it very logically, obviously, has a connection to her sex life and her sexuality and its future expression. A girl will more often than not begin to build physical and sexual relationships in the first decade after menarche, so the trouble caused by the menstrual taboo can include a negative impact on her developing sexuality, affecting the way she sees her body and what she decides to do with it.

> *I think it's as much a frontier for men as it is for women. Advertising has done much to break down the taboo of periods and feminine hygiene products, but in my experience, men still think it's some alien horror show.*

> *I am so drained by conversations with my partner where my very real feelings are dismissed for being "hormonal" and somehow less valid. While I acknowledge that my state of mind can change wildly before my period I also long to feel truly heard at these times. This is deeply complex, but I believe it's almost at the biological and spiritual heart of misogyny. I hope and aspire to my daughter and all daughters feeling less bound, less judged and less silenced than I do in this regard.*

Girls becoming women are often navigating some complex and potentially treacherous terrain as they pursue a sex life (and figure out their own sexuality), or have one projected onto them, through

> "I think it's as much a frontier for men as it is for women. Advertising has done much to break down the taboo of periods and feminine hygiene products, but in my experience **men still think it's some alien horror show.**"

partners, pornography or a vacuum created by a lack of positive sex education. It is during adolescence that young women learn the power and value of their bodies, how to listen to them, what they want from sexual interactions and how to negotiate them. These are the fundamental building blocks of bodily autonomy, which is the entitlement of every human being. But it's also the time that girls are initiated into the menstrual taboo and are taught to devalue and mistrust their bodies, leading to some long-lasting damage. The silence and stigma caused by the menstrual taboo has a number of harmful impacts on girls and women, from hurting their sense of self-respect, body image, openness and honesty with loved ones, to negatively affecting their sexual development, grasp of consent, pleasure and desire.

> *I was 20 and getting to know a nice, cute new boyfriend. One day I mentioned I had my period and he visibly cringed and said, 'Can't you just say PMS?' I was shocked and asked, 'Do you even know what that means?'. It turned out he didn't and was majorly grossed-out by periods, even the word period. Well, I won't say this was the reason we didn't last long, but it was definitely a factor. I couldn't imagine being with someone who, for five days month after month, would be disgusted by the state of my body, of me. After that I decided that whoever I was with had to be cool with periods. When I went out with my husband on our first date I casually mentioned them, and he was relaxed and happy about engaging in period-talk. The rest is history as they say.*

A 2005 study, published in *The Journal of Sex Research*, examined the connection between menstrual shame, body anxiety and sexual decision-making. They found demonstrable links between girls and women feeling ashamed of their bodies, and what they decide to do with them, sexually. 'As expected, women who reported feeling more comfort about menstruation also reported more body comfort and, in turn, more sexual assertiveness, more sexual experience, and less sexual risk'.[ix] In 2004, researchers hypothesised that 'perhaps more than any other bodily function, menstruation must be kept "under wraps" in a sexually objectifying culture' and that 'girls' and women's feelings of acceptance for their bodily functions and physical embodiment are antithetical to "self-objectification", wherein individuals internalise an outsider's standard of physical appearance'.[x] All of which is a slightly complicated way of saying that girls can be more resistant to objectifying themselves by making peace with their menstrual cycle and learning to appreciate the complexity of their bodies.

If girls get the message that a natural process of their body is shameful, wrong and repulsive, this will obviously affect their relationship with their body, and with other people's bodies. How can girls develop a strong physical sense of themselves, if they come to understand this natural process of their body as disgusting? Tuning into the body, its desires and pleasures, its warning signs, its in-built protection mechanisms, helps girls to learn that it is valuable and unique despite its challenges. Once they accept that their body has its own value and integrity, girls can develop the skills required to really trust and care for their body. If they are told, for instance, that their feelings are 'just' PMS, how will they connect to the valid anger, suspicion or frustration that they sometimes feel? There are times that girls, and women, should be angry. Reducing us to 'bitchy', 'moody' 'psychos' who 'must be on that time of the month' is the taboo at work, invalidating and gaslighting women.[xi]

We want girls to have all the facts they need to make good decisions, but we also need them to make friends with their body and take ownership of it as something worth protecting and honouring. If a girl does not think her body is worth anything, why would she expect others to treat it like it was? What is she likely to think of other women's bodies? How will she learn what her body is capable of if she does not know what its constitutive parts are there for, or even what they're called?

If a woman is alienated from her body, and does not see the value in it, and actually sees it as something gross and something that is letting her down, will she respect that body? Will she expect others to respect her body? Will she treat it as something worthwhile, worthy of protecting and nourishing; keeping it safe and healthy? The menstrual taboo can prevent women from understanding that their body has its own sovereignty and integrity. It also stops them from starting a lifelong relationship with their body that is characterised by respecting, understanding and valuing it for the right reasons.

Our bodies house us, get us where we need to go, and connect us to our loved ones (sometimes even creating them!) – that is more important than what it looks like or who is turned on by it. Girls and women on the path to that knowledge can lose their way in the shadow of the menstrual taboo.

The experience of menopause can also be very confronting and distressing for some women, especially if they don't fully understand the biological process their body is going through, as many of our respondents both expressed and regretted. There are side effects of menopause that can directly impact on a woman's sexual experience, including things like sleeplessness, night sweats, vaginal dryness and thinning of the vaginal walls, but her whole life may be impacted in measurable ways.

> *When I was exhausted from waking and hot flushing every night for months, my now ex-husband could only be scathing and dismissive. As much as women need a great deal more information and support around menopause, men need education, so they can appreciate and understand the process, and thereby offer some support!*

Because menopause is not simply a physical process, the effects can resonate far beyond the bodily or the sexual, encompassing shifts in identity, relationships and emotional states, all of which also affect our libido. Bodies are always changing, but menopause intensifies this process, and carries such emotional and social weight. Quite apart from whether a woman feels like having sex, these effects can just be difficult to live with day-to-day. Nonetheless, there are many postmenopausal women who have active and energetic sex lives that may have changed in nature or frequency from earlier in their lives but reinforce the fact that women don't go through menopause and cease to be sexual beings. Whether or not that means that their sex drive increases, decreases, or changes, the idea that somehow the double discrimination of sex and age can result in women feeling completely desexualised, and viewed as asexual, is an unfair burden for older women to carry.

That said, many women welcome these changes and accept them as a graduation to the next phase of life. This kind of positive acknowledgment is also marginalised and little discussed. This is still the menstrual taboo at work, relaying all that judgment and stigma into the condemnation of older women as having outlived their usefulness. That can obviously have an impact on women's ability to negotiate their sexual selves, but the fact remains that the best preparation we could give women for the new frontier of menopause is a healthy, respectful view of menarche and menstruation throughout their life leading up to that point.

Conception and contraception: managing fertility under the taboo

The number of women who acknowledge a limited understanding of their fertility and menstrual cycle, is also a result of the menstrual taboo at work, contributing to real suffering and difficulty. For many women, sex and fertility are closely related. A woman might spend a decade or more making sure she does not get pregnant, before turning her attention to the opposite of contraception: conception and the ability to become pregnant and carry a child. Both realities can be emotionally and psychologically draining, as well as the many states in between; of not knowing whether reproduction is for you, or knowing for sure that is isn't, and dealing with the consequences of all your decisions (and indecision). It's a set of pressures that come with a womb – what will I do with it? I want it to stay empty. I want it to be full now. I want it to work better, to stop hurting me, to give me a break, to be my friend, to reveal its magic, to start bleeding again, to stop, to contract, to relax, to retire. Everybody who has a uterus has a relationship with it, whether they know it or not, be it positive, negative, indifferent or changeable.

Contraception is very often abstracted from this emotional dimension and is instead just a routine aspect of daily life for many. It makes sense that significant numbers of women (and men) have never even considered how it works, given the general lack of familiarity with the female reproductive system and its functions. If a woman does not know the purpose of all its parts and how they interact, managing her fertility can be a frustrating, confusing and scary process. There is a large percentage of the population that will spend decades from their adolescence into late middle-age either trying to avoid or attain pregnancy. Consider how many decisions women make to prevent and achieve pregnancy; shouldn't these be fully informed choices? Whether contraception or conception is the goal, the menstrual taboo makes it harder for women and girls to access all the facts they need to decide what's best for them.

The menstrual taboo also works its shame on menopausal women by stopping them from seeing their true power. Because despite the stigma and negativity associated with periods, menopausal women can also feel their worth and inherent value challenged once they cease to menstruate. Our culture tells women who menstruate that their body is doing something 'disgusting' and 'unhygienic', while telling menopausal/post-menopausal women that their bodies are no longer 'useful', 'vital' or 'fertile': a horrible paradox spawned by the menstrual taboo, and one that would be meaningfully challenged and resolved by a proper conception of menstrual wellbeing, and more positive, broad-based knowledge and appreciation of our reproductive systems. With much better knowledge of what was happening inside, and a positive relationship with their bodies to draw on, women going through menopause would have the opportunity to see this change as empowering and strengthening, rather than the opposite.

Working through the taboo: negotiating employment

When the menstrual taboo is operating in a workplace, it reinforces secrecy and revulsion, stifling communication between women, their colleagues, and employers. It creates conditions in workplaces in which menstruating women face fundamental discrimination. Women workers feel compelled to hide the fact that they are menstruating and are more likely to call in sick, rather than tell the truth about their situation. This was mentioned many times in the responses to our survey. This is not a matter of women choosing to be dishonest, but perhaps it's an understandable response to the pressure of the taboo. A woman is likely, for instance, to use her sick leave to manage the demands of her menstrual cycle – an absurd proposition, given it is not an illness. Because menstruation itself is not a medical condition, women should not have to go to the doctor to obtain a medical certificate, which many workers are compelled to do in order to access sick leave entitlements. Apart from the fact that the health system is burdened enough without people seeking medical certificates when they have no illness, it's an effort and expense that women shouldn't need to take on for a totally normal and predictable monthly event.

> *It's obvious when I go to the toilet every two hours to change pad or tampon that I have my period, but still it's seen as time wasting.*

> *My current boss is a woman who does not seem to have the same issues with her cycle and has even gone as far as to say that she believes that women who complain about their symptoms are just being 'lazy' or 'weak'. I don't know if this is because she hasn't experienced physical discomfort to the level that some women do (like me), or if she feels like she has had to suffer through it and so all women should. Either way it would be nice to be free of this type of attitude.*

> *I have had difficult work situations where a boss has pushed for over ten minutes to work out why I was sick, when I didn't want to use the 'female' excuse. This is the biggest challenge; how to say yes, I have my period and sometimes it really hurts and makes me feel sick. I hate being made to feel that I am an inconvenience.*

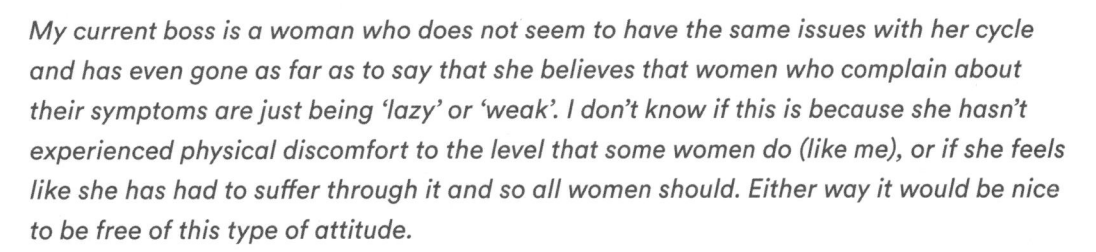

While many women have adequate facilities at their place of work, others may find that the toilets are in an area that is difficult to access or have a workplace culture that restricts their rights to access them at any time. Shift workers in retail and hospitality, for instance, may find that leaving their station during work hours is done by negotiation with managers, and this could make it harder to get to the toilet when you need to. There are many women workers who attend building sites and other outdoor or temporary workplaces, whether they are engineers, architects, construction managers, bricklayers, archaeologists, anthropologists, gardeners, landscapers, emergency service workers, road workers, truck drivers or mobile sales representatives. There might be no toilets at all, or if there are, they may not have adequate toilet paper, a bin or clean running water and soap.

Some women told us that if menstruation was referenced at all in their workplace, it was often in a negative context, including 'jokes' about PMS or menopausal maniacs, or expressing discomfort or disgust at the mention of periods or the sight of menstrual products. Others spoke candidly about feeling the need to cover up the reason for their absence from work, or of hiding periods from colleagues, slipping their tampons and pads up their sleeve before they went to the bathroom or pushing through meetings despite feeling intense pain and discomfort. It is the taboo that is causing all these women to sneak around, feeling deceitful, or gritting their teeth through the searing pain of a menstrual cramp. It's clearly unfair that women are penalised in this way through no fault of their own and this discrimination is repetitive, predictable and unacceptable.

Transforming the menstrual culture at work is about building more empathy between individuals. When empathy is a feature of a workplace, people are less likely to be reduced to one-dimensional objects, and much more likely to be viewed as fellow human beings and equals. You can imagine the impact this kind of cultural shift would have on other workplace problems, like sexual harassment and bullying. Building empathy and mutual respect is a natural inoculation against disrespect, disregard and objectification, further demonstrating the nexus of power that coalesces around shame and silence.

In her ground-breaking work on shame, Brené Brown says that the antidote is not guilt or self-love or anything you might think, but rather empathy. On shame, she says, One: we've all got it; Two: no one wants to talk about it; and Three: the less we talk about it, the more power we turn over to it, which perfectly describes the menstrual taboo. But if 'you put shame in a petri dish it needs three things to grow exponentially: secrecy, silence and judgment. If you put the same amount of shame in a petri dish and douse it with empathy it cannot survive'.[xii] (See Appendix Three for more on Brown's articulation of menstrual shame). We are burdened with all kinds of shame in our lives, but in the case of menstrual shame and the workplace, there is a clear way out, and it not only helps women but can transform workplaces into higher-functioning spaces with fewer organisational problems.

I think there is a tendency to shame women who don't disguise the fact that they are experiencing menstruation or menopause. There is also the attitude that 'hormonal' women don't function well in the work place, which makes women feel they have to hide what is happening. I once sat in a city business meeting where one of the other women apologised for the fact that I had had a hot flush then handed the decision we were making over to the only man present 'as we were all middle aged and hormonal' and she thought he would make the decision better.

Every workplace is required by law to ensure that women aren't disadvantaged by sexism, harassment, discriminatory hiring practices or because of their commitments as carers. Yet the menstrual taboo continues to facilitate this kind of discrimination. A woman writing from the UK shared her story online recently, of being sent home from the office because the hot water bottle in her lap was 'unprofessional' and had made a male colleague 'extremely uncomfortable'. The director of human resources at her workplace ordered her personally to take leave after the male co-worker complained, and she was asked 'not to disclose her medical problems to anyone who isn't part of HR as it can make them uncomfortable'.[xiii]

Or consider the case of Alisha Coleman, a 911 call taker in Georgia, USA, who was fired after ten years of service, over two incidents of sudden onset heavy bleeding, a not uncommon symptom of peri-menopause which she was experiencing at the time. After the first instance she received a warning from her employer, which cited among other complaints, that she had damaged company property (a cloth covered chair). When it happened a second time, a year later, she was fired for 'lacking high standards of cleanliness'. She engaged a lawyer but the judge in the case ruled that it was not sex discrimination. At the time of writing, the American Civil Liberties Union had taken on the case and had filed an appeal.[xiv] It was, ironically, Coleman's last period.

> *It would help if I could be late for work and not be judged for it. Some mornings when I have my period I really struggle to get motivated but also the pain makes it almost impossible to walk to work. Sometimes I need an hour to sit on the couch with a heat pack and wait for the Panadol to kick in, so I can get going.*

> *I have suffered painful periods for years due to endometriosis and at times I've had to make excuses for sick leave at work due to intense pain. In previous workplaces I've been made to feel like a whinger, with unsolicited comments about making up excuses to take time off and not being able to handle a simple period.*

> *During menopause there were days at work when I nearly passed out, and my colleagues just laughed.*

The women we spoke to often found their workplaces hostile terrain for navigating the reality of their menstrual life. The repetitive struggle of managing leave entitlements was mentioned, and having to euphemise menstrual and menopausal issues as appointments, ailments and 'sickness', among women who would much rather have honest conversations with their employers. If more workplaces reviewed their practices with a view to better accommodating employees who menstruate, or had a menstrual policy in place, it would signal to women on staff that they are respected and trusted, that having a period was not just okay but considered normal, and that the workplace was serious about supporting women. Surely an atmosphere of more openness, honesty and trust in the workplace would have to be good for business. Considering the costs shouldered by employers when turnover is high, loyalty is low, recruitment is never-ending, and training is constant; it makes sense to look at meaningful ways to help employees feel seen, heard and valued.

> I have suffered painful periods for years due to endometriosis and at times I've had to make excuses for sick leave at work due to intense pain. In previous workplaces **I've been made to feel like a whinger,** with unsolicited comments about making up excuses to take time off and not being able to handle a simple period.

Navigating the health care system: the taboo works on patients and providers

The healthcare system in Australia is envied around the world for its commitment to equality, access and universal coverage. While it may shine by comparison to other countries, we can still observe failings in the overall attitude to menstruation, menopause and assisting patients with menstrual dysfunction. Now that so many women interact with the medical system to manage their periods, fertility and its logical end, we might properly expect that women would be encouraged to learn about their cycles, know what is going on every month and trust their bodies. However, this is not the case. Not only do many women lack basic knowledge of their reproductive systems, but also the medical system is, in many instances, woefully inadequate in this sense too.

The menstrual taboo leads to disconnection and unease, for both patients and practitioners, because we lack a shared language for talking openly and constructively about menstruation. If a woman is presenting to a medical professional and cannot say what is normal for her and her cycle, this is a serious diagnostic problem. But if the same provider is also unaware of the importance of the cycle, its connection to overall health, and has no concept of menstrual wellbeing, we have a situation where both parties are severely hampered in having the kind of honest, open conversation that medical care requires. When the cultural norms of our society make women and girls feel awkward and embarrassed about taking menstrual issues to doctors, and doctors themselves can be unaware and uninformed, this impacts negatively on women's health as a field.

> *The doctors I've encountered seem to think women have no idea when their bodies are behaving inappropriately. I was told it was normal to pass golf-ball sized clots six times an hour for days on end. I was told the only 'cure' for a tipped uterus, which caused me extreme back pain, was a hysterectomy. I was told I was just imagining how bad it was. I was so frustrated that the people I went to for help didn't believe me or take me seriously, or when they did they had no idea how to actually help.*

There are also public health implications when women feel discomfited or ashamed to openly discuss their menstrual cycle with medical professionals. If women feel as though they cannot precisely or comfortably describe their cycle, its nature or symptoms of dysfunction, this has far-reaching effects. It is broadly accepted that women are vulnerable to extreme body-image issues from a young age, and that this affects their view of themselves, but it is less often explored that a basis for this might be the menstrual taboo. It is important to see the big picture here, and the connection between women's body-anxiety, the menstrual taboo and the impact on their access to medical treatment and proper health care. Dr Luci McGovern explains it succinctly: 'working extensively in the field of Obstetrics and Gynaecology I've been struck by the number of women with serious body image issues. This sense of shame is pervasive, and the scale of it to my mind constitutes a public health problem'.[xv] Until women and girls are presenting to doctors with their own knowledge and finding that medical professionals are also educated and informed, we will continue to see this public health crisis unfold.

But it is important for us to remember that menstruation is not an illness. It is not a disease, or an ailment, or even a medical condition. It is a biological process that occurs in the body spontaneously to accomplish certain physical goals. When we menstruate, our bodies are behaving exactly as they should, releasing their monthly preparation for the possible pregnancy that guarantees the continuation of the species. For the reproductive system, pregnancy is the aim, which is not necessarily consonant with our own personal choices, identity and consciousness. We can reasonably expect most uteruses, ovaries, fallopian tubes and vaginas to behave in similar ways. Endometrium will build and exit, build and exit, in a pattern that we can usually predict. There are good reasons why the menstrual cycle is a predictor and gauge of optimal physical health, as it works in concert with multiple other systems in the body to keep us well. Of course, there are conditions that lead to disorders of the menstrual cycle, like PCOS, fibroids, endometriosis, adenomyosis, and others. These illnesses are real and painful, but they are separate from normal menstrual cycling. Menstruation itself is not a dysfunction, or pollution, or a disorder (even if it sometimes feels that way), and we should resist being encouraged to view it as such.

> *A lot of people don't believe in period pain and think it's an excuse. It makes me want to bring a sledgehammer down on their pelvis.*

Despite this, women are increasingly encouraged by the medical system to interrupt their menstruation, even when it is healthy and normal. Hormonal contraceptives – the Pill, IUDs, implants, injections, vaginal rings, and skin patches all contain very similar synthetic hormones – are a common way for women to manage their fertility, but they are also chosen for non-contraceptive reasons: to suppress ovulation and make periods disappear. This is a function of the menstrual taboo producing new cultural norms around women and contraceptive drugs. A woman may find over the course of her menstruating life that she is offered medication to regulate her period, to make it disappear, to boost her fertility when she wants to conceive, and then again when she reaches menopause, to replace the ebbing hormones and mask the symptoms of her body going through such a massive change. When we look at it this way, it is disquieting to think that menstruation has become so medicalised, when for thousands of years healthy women have experienced menarche, menstruation, conception and menopause without the use of drugs.

It raises the bigger question of the medicalisation of women's bodies and the multiple and complex ways that the medical system tells us we are a set of problems to be fixed. The menstrual taboo produces and reinforces the power of these ideas, in part by limiting women's knowledge of their own biology and thus capacity for informed choice. From pregnancy and birth, to acne and hair growth, to contraception, menstruation, menopause, weight management, and even depression, women are told in various ways: 'there is something wrong with you but if you spend this money on this product, this drug, this procedure, we can fix it and in doing so fix you'. It sounds vaguely sinister when expressed this way, but it has proven to be an effective and sophisticated system of undermining and destabilising women. We might call it a gendered medical-industrial complex.

Women's health is about more than just medicine. It encompasses physical health, and treating illness and disease, of course, but it also includes emotional and psychological health, sexual health and reproduction, her place within the community, and her right to live in safety and dignity. These are not always the concerns of corporations, or even the medical system.

Pharmaceutical companies obviously have a massive impact on the medical community and which drugs are prescribed for which conditions. It's hard to think of a better drug product than the Pill for pharmaceutical companies. It is prescribed to patients who are perfectly healthy, and sometimes even for reasons not related in any way to its original stated purpose of birth control. This is referred to as 'off-label prescribing', where medicine is prescribed to patients for uses other than the purpose approved by drug regulators, which doctors are perfectly able to do legally. It is mostly prescribed to women when they are in their teens and forming their ideas about health care, medicine and medication, as well as being an age when they are less likely to challenge or refuse the recommendation. They may then take this drug, every day, for possibly decades, refilling prescription after prescription, often without anyone seriously reviewing their use of it, and they will pay for this 'peace of mind'. Blood clots, lowered libido, nausea, and even heightened risk of stroke are side-effects of the Pill that are little discussed, along with depression, anxiety and migraine. The full list includes mood swings, breast pain or tenderness, breast enlargement, fungal infections and cystitis, stomach problems and diarrhoea, irregular bleeding, skin rash and acne, hair loss, weight gain, weight loss, high or low blood pressure levels, and an inability to use contact lenses. Why do we tolerate it? The menstrual taboo is relevant here, in that it inhibits women's questions, restricts research and development in the area, and stymies demands for a better solution.

> *My daughter had very heavy periods in a stressful year of her life. She was put on two sorts of Pill. One made her weepy and unhappy, the other she had to be taken off of as she became light sensitive and had double vision – they thought it might be a blood clot. She cured herself by exercise, yoga and the gym, and by changing her diet and getting off the computer more often. I was furious that the medical system pops young women on the Pill without first considering a holistic approach.*

Many of our respondents reported their struggle with side-effects as a result of hormonal contraception, and despite being told otherwise they are not imagining it. The results of a 2016 study conducted by the University of Copenhagen of more than one million women over the course of 13 years confirmed a significant link between hormonal contraceptives and depression.[xvi] They found that use of hormonal contraception, especially among adolescents, was associated with subsequent use of antidepressants and a first diagnosis of depression, suggesting depression as a potential adverse effect of hormonal contraceptive use. Researchers found that women overall were 20 per cent more likely to be prescribed antidepressants if they had previously used hormonal contraceptives. For adolescent girls, that figure almost doubled and for the same cohort using certain LARCs (long-acting reversible contraceptives that are non-oral, such as implants and injections), the risk tripled. This confirms what many women experience, and if we consider how young many are when they begin using these drugs, it seems unbelievable that we haven't interrogated these cultural norms further. The taboo works to prevent open discussion about these important decisions in the lives of women and girls and circumscribes the conversations we have with medical professionals about our bodies and our physical needs. Dismantling the taboo would mean that girls and women making such crucial choices about what they put in their bodies could do so from a position of knowledge and familiarity with their cycle. Certainly, most women and girls make these decisions within complicated social and cultural structures, including gender, class, disability, race and occupation and they make their selection based on the information they have, the advice they receive, the possibilities open to them and the particular pressures they face. Undoubtedly, they do their best, but they might be able to do better in a genuine culture of informed consent and best practice among medical professionals.

But the Pill is a drug with such a strong emotional and political narrative surrounding it; related so closely to personal and gendered liberation, that sustained critique of it is often obstructed, which also benefits the companies that sell it. The manufacturers are also strongly advantaged by the common advice of GPs; that if a particular brand of the Pill produces unacceptable side effects, you should try another and another, and shop around until 'the right one' is found. Companies will develop, push and advertise variations as especially good at solving problems like acne, weight gain, loss of libido (all symptoms of the drugs themselves) at a higher price, with the same basic ingredients slightly rearranged. The Pill and LARCs have similar active ingredients, synthetic oestrogen and progesterone, or synthetic progesterone alone, but proponents of the latter argue that, in the case of hormone-releasing IUDs, the insertion of the device directly into your uterus allowing direct absorption means that a smaller dose is required for birth control purposes. It's important to note here that to do their job these hormonal mimics need to lock onto our hormone receptor sites to trigger the required reproductive interventions. The other, less widely known, design criteria is that these chemicals also need to be sufficiently different to our natural hormones to be patentable, and therefore profitable, by the pharmaceutical companies producing them.

There is also the inconvenient truth that those using the Pill may also suffer predictable side effects, like depression or weight gain, that will precipitate their use of other drugs sold by the same company, for example, anti-depressants or weight loss drugs, that are also taken daily and produce strong emotional connections and feelings of dependence. Hormonal contraception has a captive audience, including women who are terrified of getting pregnant in a society that may not respect their need to terminate, or if possible and legal, may be financially prohibitive. Not that the Pill can guarantee contraception (with a user effectiveness rate of around 92 per cent) and even the higher effectiveness of LARCS is compromised by their relatively high rate of discontinuation.[xvii]

Obviously, the field of reproductive rights is complex and brutally contested, with many women around the world totally denied formal access to the knowledge and tools they need to control their fertility. But we cannot let that reality stop us from soberly discussing another one: that the widespread prescription of hormonal contraceptives, including LARCs, to healthy girls and women should be interrogated and unpacked. At least we have the right to demand that women and girls be fully informed, about their options and the reality of risks and side effects. Women and girls should not be pressured to stay on the Pill or given false information about more or less invasive methods, because this ultimately robs them of their agency and dignity. We are all entitled to contraceptive literacy and the stakes are obviously especially high for anyone who can become pregnant. If instead we trusted and respected women to manage their own bodies and fertility, by making sure they had all the knowledge they needed, we would be contributing to a culture of empowerment and equality.

The reverse of this is the reluctance of the medical system, and many doctors within it, to listen to women and believe them when they describe what they think is wrong with their own bodies. The average time women were delayed in receiving a positive diagnosis for endometriosis is seven to twelve years, according to Endometriosis Australia. Years of excruciating pain, an inability to stand and walk in some cases, a seriously compromised quality of life, because doctor after doctor tells them that 'a bit of pain is normal' and won't believe them when they say that what they experience is debilitating and wrong.

> *I used to dread getting my period, due to pain and poor understanding of what periods were all about. But in my early twenties it became very irregular and I discovered that I had PCOS. I found a naturopath and a chiropractor who were able to help me and over time I was able to heal my ovaries and hormonal imbalance. I now have a regular 28-day cycle, though in truth I'm constantly working hard on my health in order to keep PCOS at bay, which includes being conscious of my emotions and my thoughts and how they affect my body and hormones. All this has been both a blessing for the self-awareness and personal growth this journey has taken me on, and a curse too for the constant attention I have to give it.*

'The girl who cried pain: The bias against women in the treatment of pain', a paper written by Professors Diane E. Hoffman and Anita J. Tarzian, explores this phenomenon in detail, demonstrating with evidence that not only do women feel more pain, more often (as a result of a complex interplay of hormones and physiological differences between men's and women's brains) but also that 'women who seek help are less likely than men to be taken seriously when they report pain and are less likely to have their pain adequately treated.'[xviii] One of the many reasons advanced for why this is so concerns women's superior ability to reason through pain and use better coping mechanisms and a greater repertoire of skills to manage their pain, including seeking support, both social and medical. As ever, we excel despite our difficult position.

> *I really loathe and despise the prevalent discourse around 'PMS' and the suggestion that it is a mental pathology, like in the Diagnostic and Statistical Manual of Mental Disorders Fifth Edition or DSM-V. It seems as though 'PMS' is another 'flaw' that keeps women somehow at a lower level than 'rational', 'non-cyclical' men in the very patriarchal medical and mental-health profession discourse.*

> *It's annoying how sometimes before menstruating I feel sad and angry and my mood changes drastically. I feel I lack education on the subject and I don't know how to control it. It makes me mad.*

Most women have at some time experienced the symptoms of PMS, which is unsurprising given that they include depressed mood, anxiety, irritability, bloating, tender breasts, and tiredness. Our data reflects the pressure this puts on women at certain times of the month, not only to manage these symptoms but also to conceal them (the latter of which can contribute to the aforementioned anxiety). A recent study focused on 60 women who self-identified as 'PMS sufferers' and analysed the similarities in their coping mechanisms. The researchers found that all the women's strategies fell into three categories: self-awareness, self-care, and the positive engagement of other people in their lives as a means of alleviating stress and conflict.[xix] Put simply, they found that women can cope on their own really well, by listening to their needs and meeting them, but they will cope better if they can also enlist the help of others, especially those close to them. The fantastic thing about this research is the conclusion that while women have agency and power in their own right, it is enhanced and strengthened through cooperation and openness. This is the opposite of how the taboo can isolate and disempower women.

The aforementioned study also found that women are far less likely to have their pain treated aggressively when they come into contact with medical professionals, compared with men. While men are more likely to receive analgesics as pain relief, women are more likely to receive sedatives, based on the belief that their pain is psychosomatic and will abate when they 'calm down'. Now consider what happens when that pain is related to a taboo subject. Women must first overcome their own reluctance to talk openly and honestly about their menstrual cycle, periods, flow, vagina, vulva, and uterus – not subjects that women are encouraged to feel confident discussing, even with a medical professional. Now factor in the discomfort, judgment and stigma being triggered in the attending doctor, and we can begin to imagine how the menstrual taboo might affect the fair, respectful and effective treatment of women presenting with pain related to menstrual dysfunction, and the tragedy and injustice of that.

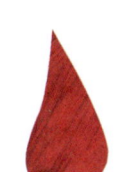

Menstrual dysfunction: worse for women as long as the taboo operates

Menstrual dysfunction is real. Many women don't even realise they suffer from one of these conditions and simply endure decades of pain and suffering. As we learn about our periods under the taboo this means that we are more likely to have a negative view of them, and be less able to develop the intimate knowledge, and awareness of our own individual cycle, required to judge our menstrual health. If a woman knows what her 'normal' is then she is much more able to tell what symptoms are 'abnormal'. Likewise, if all girls and women knew more about menstruation in general, and about other people's experience of it, they would have more reliable and beneficial gauges to measure their own menstrual wellbeing and could also help each other.

Menstrual dysfunction can be painful and debilitating, and it is very easy to see why the period itself could be seen as the cause, when the reality is that the condition, and not the period, is to blame for pain and discomfort. It makes sense that people who suffer through their period every month would be tempted to remove it altogether, but this would simply remove a symptom and not the cause. In some cases, the menstrual dysfunction holds clues that relate to your whole-body health and a holistic approach would form the basis of an effective concept of menstrual wellbeing.

> *I thought that excruciating monthly pain was normal. During my teen years I suffered such horrific cramps and heavy periods. It was my normal, but I didn't know that there was any other way to have a period I didn't know what normal was. I wish my endometriosis had been diagnosed then and I may not have lost so many years in this agonising twilight zone.*

The American College of Obstetricians and Gynaecologists recommends that physicians consider the menstrual cycle as a vital sign of overall health in adolescents.[xx] This means that along with blood pressure, breathing, temperature and pulse, it is also crucial to consider the nature of each woman's cycle as an important predictor of her physical health. In some cases, the symptoms of the menstrual dysfunction are indicators of issues with general health, including hormonal imbalances that may manifest at various times during the menstrual cycle. Treating the body holistically is a driving philosophy of many non-Western disciplines including traditional Chinese medicine and Ayurveda, as well as underpinning complementary medicine like osteopathy and naturopathy. By contrast, Western medicine tends to view medical issues in isolation and works from the premise of removing the symptoms of dysfunction locally and directly. Obviously, people want their pain treated and removed, and doctors may well be acting with compassion, but there is also a bigger question of how we analyse chronic issues and approach our health care holistically. While there is obviously a place for both approaches, menstrual health is particularly ill-served by being viewed in isolation.

In a matter of decades, we have moved to a new paradigm of medicalising menstruation, offering women quick fixes, drugs, medical treatment, menstrual suppression, and expensive (sometimes harmful) products, to make our bleeding minimal, invisible or cease altogether. If this is our best offer to women experiencing painful or heavy periods, or secondary dysmenorrhea (endometriosis and PCOS commonly) then we have serious work to do. We need to move beyond a paradigm of reflexively recommending LARCs and surgery to women experiencing menstrual dysfunction and provide genuine information about less invasive alternatives whereever possible. We need a medical system with better responses to these conditions, but we also need better treatments. We need more research and more funding. The pervasiveness of the menstrual taboo means that women and girls all too often don't get proper care and early intervention.

When women do experience pain every month around their periods, the message is usually to manage it and keep quiet about it, with the menstrual taboo preventing many women from speaking openly about their situation and needs. The reality is that if we had a more functional and open dialogue around menstruation, it would be possible for more women to gauge what level of pain is reasonable and what is not. Too often this process is drawn out and protracted because women feel dismissed, or because they are told directly that they are imagining the distress, that the pain is normal, that they need to work it out themselves. As reflected in our data, many women who report menstrual dysfunction to medical practitioners are often given very few options. Some are told 'it's in your head', that they are imagining it and to change their way of thinking in order to fix it. Many are urged to take the Pill or use LARCs to suppress ovulation (or get rid of the period altogether). More than one woman told us that their doctor suggested having a baby, asserting that pregnancy and childbirth will 'sort it out'. As well as being untrue for many women, the existence of this pattern points to a serious lack of understanding, denying women the right to diagnosis, treatment, dignity and respect.

One in ten Australian women suffer from endometriosis, with similar numbers among menstruating women and girls worldwide. As mentioned, the average delay in diagnosing the disease can be up to seven to twelve years. Surgery is required to diagnose endometriosis and is also a common treatment, though it does not always provide a permanent solution – the treatment for endometriosis is to track its growth and go under the knife to cut it away, or have laser treatment at regular intervals. This is what women routinely suffer and recent figures suggest that endometriosis affects around 600,000 Australian women and 176 million women worldwide.[xxi] This is not a small problem. Recently, in Australia we have seen serious funding and political will directed at endometriosis research, treatment and education through the National Action Plan for Endometriosis (2018), which is excellent, but it bears thinking about why it took so long to see this action materialise. Surely, we can accept that it is partly due to the fact that it is women who suffer through it, largely in silence, and that it relates to a stigmatised process. The menstrual taboo has contributed to this dangerous indifference for too long, and it is the loosening of its grip that has allowed meaningful attention to be garnered.

Polycystic ovarian syndrome affects twelve to eighteen per cent of Australian women of reproductive age and up to 21 per cent in some high-risk groups such as Indigenous women.[xxii] It is discovered and diagnosed by ultrasound and CAT scan and ongoing intermittent surgical treatment is usually required. Fibroids are another common affliction among menstruating women and while many of them are benign, in some cases they can affect fertility and cause pain and other symptoms. We heard from one woman who saw a doctor for acute, chronic pain related to her fibroids. He suggested that she could 'just have a hysterectomy since you've already had children so it won't matter'. She sought a second opinion and the next doctor advised her to manage the pain with paracetamol, which she found to be woefully inadequate. This story, in microcosm, reflects how many women experience the health care system when they present with menstrual dysfunction; inconsistency and lack of knowledge, and the dismissal of chronic pain as simply something women should tolerate.

If so many women suffer these kinds of afflictions and they are chronically under-diagnosed and treated, what does this tell us? Why don't we have better funding and treatments for these conditions? How can women live for years in extreme and chronic pain, with their whole lives constrained by their menstrual cycle, and not be believed when they ask for help? These are not small problems. They represent serious failures in the health care system and point to the menstrual taboo at work. The pressure this puts on women to carry on, regardless of pain and suffering, is unfair and unreasonable. Whether your menstruation is normal or dysfunctional the menstrual taboo makes it harder, and limits your options for managing fertility, your cycle and its cessation at menopause.

Something else we might consider is that as long as the medical and scientific communities treat the menstrual cycle as mysterious, irrelevant or simply without interest we are missing out on important discoveries that could revolutionise our lives. You might know that stem cells – the extremely valuable immature cells found in the umbilical cord blood of newborns, are the building blocks of regenerative medicine. Harvesting stem cells is generally painstaking and difficult, but did you know that the endometrium also contains stem cells? Neither did anybody else until early this century.[xxiii] That stuff we throw away, put inside chemical bins and generally find disgusting and revolting? It could be a major source of stem cells that does not need to be invasively harvested. What other secrets are contained within our cycles? Are we really so surprised that an environment that can build human beings from scratch is medically and scientifically significant in the extreme? The sooner we pull apart the menstrual taboo and liberate our scientific imaginations about the menstrual cycle, the more ground-breaking enquiry can enlarge our understandings of life itself and women's centrality to it.

Hip pocket penalties: the taboo forcing Australian women to pay and pay

Right now, in Australia, there are more commercial products available to manage menstruation than at any time before, including those that can be conveniently ordered online and shipped from overseas. Most Australian women use a combination of single use, disposable items: tampons, pads and panty liners. Other products gaining popularity include menstrual cups, period underwear, and reusable cloth pads. How many women try these alternatives, and whether they discover them at all, is often circumscribed by the taboo and its effects on our beliefs around hygiene, propriety and safety. If you believe, or were raised to think, that putting your fingers inside your vagina is wrong, then this may affect your choice of menstrual product. Similarly, if you are repulsed by the sight of menstrual blood and find it unseemly to look at it or touch it, you might also choose products that help you avoid it as much as possible.

Consider too the very fact that we call menstrual products 'sanitary items' and talk about 'feminine hygiene', along with myriad other euphemisms for everything from our periods to the supplies we use to manage them. Different cultural contexts may approach menstruation in markedly different ways, but these terms have become near universal. Many women labour under the illusion that this means their tampons and pads are sterile, like a bandage or syringe, but they are much more like toilet paper or tissues in terms of their production and packaging. In some parts of the world it may be necessary, in a development context, to speak about menstrual hygiene where there is limited access to amenities and water. But the persistent use of words like 'sanitary' and 'hygiene' in Australian classrooms and supermarket aisles represents a failure of precision and clarity. There is no need to euphemise periods, menstruation, tampons, pads or any other product, and the insistence on it harks back to more conservative times when advertisers needed to work around the taboo. It is this triumph of marketing jargon and a reluctance to speak openly about menstruation that has produced linguistic and cognitive dissonance, and it does not help women and girls to think of their periods as unhygienic or unsanitary.

Our survey showed that the politics of these products are deeply felt and observed by the women who use and choose them. Some talked about their reluctance to use tampons because their mothers had forbidden them, to protect their modesty and virginity. Another woman recounted being ridiculed by a colleague for asking to borrow a pad when she got caught out by her period: 'Who uses pads!' she said, the implication being that it was wrong, unfashionable or unhygienic to do so. Sadly, women and girls policing each other is one of the effects of patriarchy, and in the case of menstruation, this occurs within a matrix of shame, stigma, fear and reproach.

It is not what kind of products you use – as these will always be different to someone else's choice – but rather the taboo at work, making people not only feel embarrassed or ashamed by their choices at times, but feeling defensive or the need to assert superiority over others. In the absence of a menstrual taboo, women and girls would not only see more options available to them in the marketplace and in educational settings, but they might talk more openly and constructively among themselves about the best thing for managing their period.

Disposable tampons and pads have different associations and overtones to many of the women who use them, but their introduction in Australia heralded decisive and very real freedoms. Replacing torn cloths strips (rags) in the case of working-class women, and expensive, uncomfortable and unwieldy harnesses and belts among the more privileged, the disposability of pads and tampons was the very height of modern sophistication and welcomed by women as a liberating and convenient solution to an age-old problem.

From their inception tampons have been connected to nascent waves of female independence and freedom, coming to prominence as they did after French nurses innovated with absorbent bandages during World War I. By World War II, advertisers were keen to exploit the new desire women had for convenience, invisibility (when wearing slacks!) and the ability to 'soldier on' regardless of the period. There was explicit linking of competence and independence with tampon use and despite the early and obvious focus on middle class, married women, the association with modernity and liberation persisted. It also meant connecting the convenience and cleanliness of single use disposables to strong women who are in charge of themselves and their destiny, in a sleight of hand with huge implications for the environment, large-scale sanitation systems and the hip pocket of women everywhere.

Tampons, of course, were at the centre of a large-scale breakdown of safety for women users, when they were positively linked to Toxic Shock Syndrome (TSS) in the 1980s and 1990s.[xxiv] In the US, the crisis was connected to a popular line of ultra-absorbent tampons, which were not accompanied by sufficient information for the women using them, and who were encouraged to rely on them for long periods without changing. Research also pointed to the synthetic materials that were increasingly used at the time, including manufactured cellulose fibres like rayon, as well as bleaches like dioxin. Though the development of the disease is complicated, the outbreak of TSS cases and their link to tampon use highlights the unique problem of menstrual products that interface with the body in this way – they are generally not classified as medical products, which are governed by strict laws regarding development, access, disclosure, instructions, manufacture and sale. They are treated by most governments as cosmetic or luxury items, or not regulated at all. America brought them under the jurisdiction of the FDA (Food and Drug Administration) in the 1980s, and in Australia, they are classified under the Therapeutic Goods Act 1989, which requires that they are produced, labelled and sold displaying specific information. This is good but there have also been genuine concerns raised about the manufacturing processes of these products, including the chemicals used to treat the materials, and the actual ingredients used.

If the average woman who uses tampons can spend 100,000 hours of her life with one inserted, this is a reasonable question for women, in every country, to want answered. The vagina is a particularly sensitive and moist part of the body so if we use products that are produced with bleach, fragrance and other chemicals we need to be conscious of that. Added to this vaginal fluid, which helps to maintain healthy pH balance and guard against infection, is soaked up by tampons not able to discriminate between menstrual blood and vaginal secretions. The absorbency of tampons also presents problems for waste disposal and environmental impact, and the plastic used in pads and panty liners takes between 500 and 800 years to degrade in landfill, but the menstrual taboo diminishes our capacity to have open and frank discussions about this.[xxv]

> *Now I use a menstrual cup and I like seeing the colour and amount of my menstrual blood. I feel it gives me an increased awareness of my body.*

> *Menstruation has become more meaningful for me since having children and since using my own home-made pads. I feel more connected with my body and the broader cycle of life, and it's helped me embrace my womanhood.*

> *It's been wonderful to come to a different appreciation of menstruation. I use cloth pads to reduce the skin irritation I get from disposables. In the last few years my yearning to make it a positive experience for my daughter has enabled this transformation for me. I feel much more whole somehow now.*

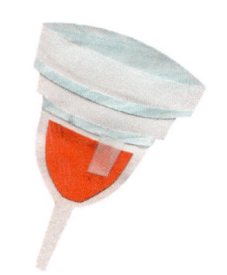

And therein lies another quandary – there is no doubt that the introduction of disposable pads and tampons did revolutionise women's lives at a time when the alternatives available may have felt limiting and restrictive or were less appealing. There is no doubt that the rise of disposables, and the later addition of an adhesive strip to pads, changed many women's experience of their period for the better. It is worth noting that these products were for a long time accessible only to middle class and well-off women, and that the expansion of their reach to less affluent women was also highly significant (period poverty notwithstanding). This isn't to say that women shouldn't use tampons! Just that in the absence of a taboo, women may have more consumer choice in managing their periods, and they may feel more comfortable and entitled to demand more information about the manufacturing and materials of these products. We might have considered the environmental impact of using these products sooner and felt more comfortable using a mix of different methods to manage our periods.

Menstrual cups are a big part of this shift in demand for more environmentally friendly alternatives to managing periods. Though only accounting for a small percentage of the market to date, there is an increased interest in how cups can transform the experience of menstruating for the better and focus groups have found high satisfaction rates among people who try a cup to manage their period. A study conducted by the Vancouver Island Women's Clinic in Canada in 2011 found that women who typically used tampons but switched to menstrual cups for three months reported higher satisfaction with their period product than those who continued to use tampons, particularly in regard to convenience and leakage. And 91 per cent of the participants said they would continue to use the cup and would recommend it to others.[xxvi] Of course, as a concept, they still struggled

" A doctor told me when I was a teenager that my period pain would go away once I had children. Now at 47 I'm still spending money on tampons, pain relief and psych visits for PMS. I wonder how much better we could manage periods if the serious needs of **half the human race** were given the equivalent funding to male impotence or the military. "

with the elements of the taboo that are reinforced and upheld by disposable single-use product advertising – that women and girls shouldn't interact with their menstrual blood, or have too much familiarity between their fingers and their vagina, and that it would be somehow unhygienic and unsanitary to reuse a recyclable product. These ideas also work against reusable cloth pads and period underwear, which are both better for the environment and cheaper in the long run. Attitudes are certainly changing but while the menstrual taboo is upheld and reinforced in so many parts of our society (including through advertising), thoughtful conversations about different products, and more choice, will be slow and painstaking.

Top-down taboo: taxing your non-essential period products

Did you know that until recently there was a GST (Goods and Services Tax) charged on your tampons, pads and panty liners? You probably did because you signed a dozen petitions to have it removed. Many efforts were made here in Australia to change the taxation status of menstrual products, with every campaign until 2018 having failed. It has been a longstanding and slow-burning issue for activists who have tried many different strategies to see the tax lifted. Intermittently a politician would pick up the issue, introduce a private members bill, or add it to a raft of legislation, to address it. The successful bill was ultimately introduced by Senator Janet Rice of The Greens, but the removal of the tax had broad support across all major parties.

Axing the so-called tampon tax has strong support among Australian women, and many men, but not everyone knows the story behind it and how we came to accept an extra financial penalty just for managing our periods.

> *A doctor told me when I was a teenager that my period pain would go away once I had children. Now at 47 I'm still spending money on tampons, pain relief and psych visits for PMS. I wonder how much better we could manage periods if the serious needs of half the human race were given the equivalent funding to male impotence or the military.*

When the Goods and Services Tax was introduced by the Howard government in 2000, John Howard was adamant that no goods or services would be exempt. The Democrats in the Senate demurred, and because they held the balance of power, were able to force the issue and give most fresh food, medical supplies, and other essentials a special status. That word, essentials, is very important here.

There's something very interesting coalescing around a debate of what is considered 'essential'. Menstruation is indisputably an essential part of life. It is essential that we support those who menstruate so that they can be productive, healthy members of society, but also so that human life can continue. This essential quality of menstruation is what is denied by the taboo, and in refusing to recognise the vital nature of the products we use to manage it, the state participates directly in the undermining and devaluing of this fundamental and natural process. The state creates a reality for everyone who lives under it but is not itself a fixed and objective reality.

Rather it is created through the prism of male experience and is an expression of patriarchal power. Because menstruation largely falls outside the direct experience and purview of men, it can be relegated, othered and seen as separate to the whole (or the norm), when in fact it is central to our existence. We discussed patriarchal systems earlier, and the state – its instrumentalities, culture and systematic application of the rule of law – was built on masculinist approaches and perspectives. It also reflects male anxieties. What men don't experience or fully grasp is so often assigned the status of irrelevant or unimportant.

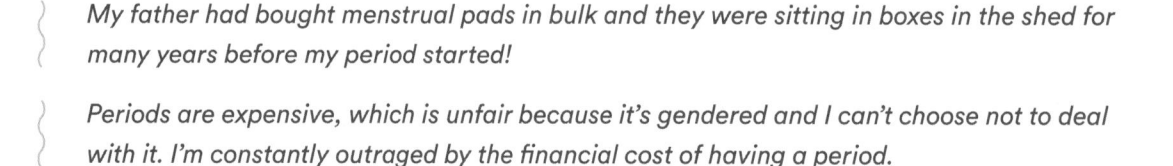

> *My father had bought menstrual pads in bulk and they were sitting in boxes in the shed for many years before my period started!*
>
> *Periods are expensive, which is unfair because it's gendered and I can't choose not to deal with it. I'm constantly outraged by the financial cost of having a period.*
>
> *Please stop the awful fragrance ads, which make people think that 'down there' is an ugly or unclean place.*

If we accept – as the government of the day certainly did and successive governments have held the line – that certain items are essential, and so important to public amenity, health and safety, that they should be exempted from a tax that classes them among luxuries, why didn't menstrual products qualify? Sunscreen did. Condoms and lubricant did. Incontinence pads are exempt. There is a discernible pattern here.

All these items are agreed to be essential in maintaining public standards of health, dignity and wellbeing, for all people. It is absurd that similar items, essential to the health, dignity and wellbeing of half the population, were not treated the same way, and made easier for people to access. Was it harder for the politicians in the room to argue this case robustly amongst male peers? Did the general embarrassment people feel at talking about tampons and pads affect the negotiations for exemptions?

Could it be that because these products are for women, specifically for menstruation, that successive governments could continue to discriminate against us for decades? Almost certainly it's the menstrual taboo in action that stopped women from more effectively agitating against this absurd inequality. But because menstruation is not a part of men's lived experience, and they are often in the positions of authority and control over these policies, the taboo works on them also. Efforts were undertaken, petitions signed, fusses well and truly kicked up, and yet here we are, almost two decades after the introduction of the GST only just having had this rectified.

Not only are women still paid significantly less for doing the same job, we also have to fork out for pads and tampons, pain relief and replacement underwear, clothes and linen – not to mention footing the bill for contraception and on government luxury tax! These things are a substantial and all too regular cost, especially if you bleed heavily and long like some. Periods should be considered a service performed for society.

We paid a tax on tampons, which was unfair, but this financial penalty pales into insignificance when we consider what we pay in so many other ways because of the menstrual taboo: culturally, socially, psychologically and individually. What is this really costing us? Women have told us what it costs them personally, and as a society it is costing us too.

Taboo or not taboo, that is the question

'One of the reasons taboos die so hard – in all types of civilisations – is that they are rigorously taught to youngsters, who dare not question them. To the uninitiated, they represent the status and privilege of adulthood.' [xxvii]

We know some taboos exist for very good reasons. Many are upheld and observed because the benefits are so clear and obvious that the costs are easily outweighed. Others are perpetuated for the sake of tradition, remaining in place because they go largely unexamined. All taboos have one thing in common: they rise and fall based on the number of people who consider them worth keeping. They are not natural or immutable laws. They are developed by societies and cultures in order to protect what is valued or sacred to the group, and they are often self-explanatory.

But what about those taboos that are confounding, confusing or outdated?

Rational decision-making often employs the economic tool of cost-benefit analysis: a process of calculating and comparing different options available, in the interests of helping us to make the most sensible and efficient choices. When evidence suggests that costs outweigh benefits, we naturally seek to redress back to a state of balance or profit. But in the case of the menstrual taboo, do the costs outweigh the benefits? Let's put it to the test.

We need to begin by examining the benefits to maintaining the taboo. In truth, it's difficult to view them as genuinely beneficial to anyone other than a very small group of people who may profit from the continuation of menstrual shame and stigma. For instance, for those who like to maintain hierarchical relationships in the patriarchal mould, the menstrual taboo provides a type of 'proof' that women are weaker and less capable. Anyone who see periods as a particularly unpleasant necessity are benefited, in that the taboo keeps outward signs of menstruation hidden to a large extent. Arguments for better medical research, social justice, targeted education and specialist health care, about menstruation and menopause, are much harder to make in the atmosphere of the taboo, which effectively diminishes awareness and silences those who seek it. This saves money in the short term for governments, but the long-term costs will certainly mount. On a more personal level, the general discomfort and ignorance about menstruation means that some women and girls can leverage this with teachers, partners, employers, or family, to avoid things they don't want to do, without much resistance. And one real benefit of the taboo is the genuine camaraderie and support generated between women in the face of it – where women and girls overcome shame and reach out for each other; this mutual sharing can be especially joyful. These are some of the discernible benefits (such as they are) of the menstrual taboo in practice. It is a bleak view and one that is clearly reflected in our research and in the experience of so many women and girls.

Let's now examine the costs in maintaining the menstrual taboo. According to Endometriosis Australia endometriosis costs the economy more than $7 billion a year. Women as individuals can spend in the region of $20,000 over a lifetime on products to manage their periods, having also paid extra taxes. There are also the opportunity costs for women who struggle with period pain and its effect on their career prospects. Having workplaces and economic models that punish women for having menstruating bodies can result in derailment, deferment and lack of progression for women at crucial stages in their professional lives (much like the decision to have children, also related to bodies). There are aspects of women's lived experience that are simply too complex to express in dollar figures.

As with women's unpaid labour being ignored by the GDP, the costs of menstruation are often rendered invisible, which, unsurprisingly, makes hard econometric data difficult to source. Even if we had more hard statistics, they would scarcely convey the full extent of the problem we face.

Similarly, the social and emotional costs of the menstrual taboo cannot be reduced to numbers. It impacts girls and women in myriad ways, as we've seen, and has serious consequences for their future health outcomes – physical, mental and sexual – and their lifelong relationship with their body. With some girls absenting themselves from school altogether, many others will simply end their involvement in sport, with the taboo providing the perfect cover for refusing physical activity. Their quality of their educational experience is affected because they carry anxiety and negativity around them throughout the school years, though perhaps especially in the years close to menarche when they are more vulnerable. The confidence of girls falls drastically after menarche,[xxviii] with girls twice as likely as boys to suffer depression during adolescence.

Girls who become sexually active without having a strong sense of themselves, their bodies, their cycle and their fertility are at higher risk of poor sexual decision-making, sexual dissatisfaction, and even unwanted pregnancy. For women trying to conceive, being ignorant of their reproductive health and processes can bring unnecessary difficulty, and there is also a strong link between menstrual shame and traumatic birth outcomes and maternal distress. For menopausal and peri-menopausal women, a lack of preparation, awareness and options can lead to social isolation, and significant impacts on physical, mental and financial wellbeing. All these individual costs compound into far greater societal ones, considering the very real burden on families, communities, the health care system, and the economy.

From our perspective, the results are stark: the financial costs alone are immense. But what of the costs that can't be quantified – what does it cost a woman to spend her whole life disconnected from her body and not trusting its functions? Nobody can put a figure on the anxiety that girls and women carry with them, month in month out, over the course of their lives. These realities can't be reduced to sums on balance sheets.

Yet, this taboo surrounding menstruation is pervasive and costly. We are all harmed by it. Yes, even those of us who do not menstruate. Yes, even those of us who haven't started yet, or who have already finished, or who suppress their ovulation cycle to get rid of periods altogether. Yes, even those of us with non-cycling bodies, with no uterus or vagina or vulva, who have never and will never have a period. And yes, for those of us with a menstrual cycle, with a reproductive system containing ovaries, fallopian tubes, a cervix and a uterus, who get periods, who meet the blood month in and month out, who bleed and bleed, the pain we carry might be more deeply felt and more incapacitating. Suffering can't be weighed and measured and expressed as a numerical value.

The spectacular truth is that if we smashed the menstrual taboo, the benefits would be beyond any measure. We could look forward to more equal and open relationships between women and men, girls and boys, parents and children, teachers and students, employers and employees, all of which could suffuse our society with a renewed respect for women, their innate power and the integrity of their bodies. We would expect more effective contributions to the economy, better productivity and increased growth in workplaces across the country. We would significantly reduce the burden on the health care system, by seizing the opportunity to better equip women for a lifetime of interacting with their bodies from a place of knowledge and acceptance. We could expect better outcomes for women's health generally, with positive impacts for public health more broadly, and especially in the fields of reproductive and sexual health.

Pushing through the taboo

Change is definitely in the air, and our call to dismantle the menstrual taboo is empowered and emboldened by what we observe around the world – spontaneous outbreaks of menstrual positivity! People everywhere are starting to wonder why this normal and natural process has been so demonised and derided, and in some cases, they are coming up with creative and innovative ways to challenge the taboo with the counterforces of logic, compassion, care and courage.

On the workplace front, the Victorian Women's Trust (VWT) instituted a Menstrual and Menopause Wellbeing Policy in May 2016, becoming one of the first Australian organisations to do so. This initiative has been a resounding success, attracting global interest and support, with widespread coverage within Australia, Canada and France.

The rationale for the VWT's policy is as follows: Experiences of menstruation and menopause can be very debilitating, yet we have been enculturated to mask their existence in the workplace, at schools and at home. The policy supports employees in their ability to adequately self-care during their period and menopause, while not being penalised by having to deplete their sick leave. Periods and menopause are not a sickness after all. The policy also seeks to remove the stigma and taboo surrounding menstruation and menopause. The policy is designed to provide opportunities for restful working circumstances and self-care for employees experiencing symptoms of menstruation and menopause. The policy is designed to be flexible depending on the employee's needs, empowering them to manage their own wellbeing.

Initially, the younger women at the VWT were slightly bemused by the taking up of the menstrual project. But this soon changed. With the acknowledgement that menstruation was a regular occurrence and can be accompanied by cyclic emotional and physical needs staff embraced the idea of a menstrual workplace policy. Some staff realised how often they had concealed their menstruation and menopause in the past and embraced a new era of period positivity in the workplace.

One woman said, 'Once I understood what this was about I felt I was more able to be at work as my whole self, that I could be there as a menstruating woman as well, and this made everything easier.' Across the organisation, some staff had taken up options one and two without much disruption to workflow, and tellingly, less than ten days of menstrual leave were taken in total over three years.

Women at the VWT found that the Menstrual and Menopause Wellbeing Policy (See Appendix Four) made it easier and more comfortable to talk about menstruation and this in turn made it easier to be at work with menstrual symptoms or needs. By the end of the trial it was decided that the policy would offer three options; modified work environment, flexible work arrangement, and paid time off, which allowed women to choose what would help them when they were menstruating, if needed. The VWT found that the entitlements were not abused, there was a measurable and significant boost to workplace morale, and that the organisation now felt it had taken a positive step towards workplace equality for women.

At around the same time, the British company Coexist instituted a menstrual leave policy after one of its directors saw a huge gap in the way her company cared for its women employees. Bex Baxter later delivered a TED Talk called 'Ending A Workplace Taboo. Period.' explaining how one day she saw a valued company employee doubled over in visible pain, continuing to do her job. When Baxter intervened to say that the employee should go home immediately, she replied in four words that changed everything: 'It's just my period.'; a phrase that most women have uttered or heard many times in their lives, working or otherwise. It was this absurdity, this juxtaposition of the woman 'just getting on with it', in such extremis, that struck Baxter as the beginning of an opportunity to overhaul their workplace and make it genuinely accepting and supportive of its women workers.[xxix] It has certainly been the case for the women at VWT, and as more workplaces take up the opportunity, it seems certain to result in greater productivity, and greater job satisfaction, for so many women.

Menstrual activism can take so many forms, so while corporates and companies may advertise to women using feminist language, and not-for-profit organisations may lobby government directly for better solutions, individual women have made some truly excellent cultural and artistic statements in support of menstrual empowerment, and speaking out against the gender gap between those who have to manage their periods and those who benefit from women doing this in silence.

Judy Chicago's 1971 artwork, *Red Flag*, depicted a bloodied tampon being removed from a vagina hidden in shadows. It was somehow instantly iconic and iconoclastic all at once, and it ushered in a new era of confrontational feminist art, with equally radical politics and aesthetics. More recently we have seen the effort of pushing through the taboo from women like Kiran Gandhi, who bled freely while she ran the 2015 London Marathon, and Rupi Kaur, who took on Instagram over the deletion of her photographs depicting a menstrual bleed, incidentally demonstrating the leadership of women of colour on this and other feminist issues.

But some examples of menstrual activism are sweet, simple, and found in unlikely places. Male students at James Hillgrove High in New Haven, Connecticut, were so moved by the unfair expectations on their female peers, they organised a donation drive for menstrual products, and encouraged boys in the school to keep a tampon or pad on hand in case a friend ever needed one. In showing solidarity with the girls, who needed to think about this all time and make sure they always had emergency supplies stashed somewhere, the boys felt that everyone could contribute to a better environment. In a proactive step to involve everyone in a more equitable solution, they decided to share some of the responsibility for menstrual management, showing real compassion and care, but also a knack for nimble innovation.

Here in Australia, the actor and singer Lucy Peach is creating theatrical shows, presenting TED talks and developing school workshops that take a positive approach to periods. She even wrote a suite of songs to correspond with her menstrual cycle, after keeping a journal of her experiences over some months! Her Perth Fringe show 'My Greatest Period Ever' (which also had a young adult adaptation, 'How to Period Like a Unicorn') features a combination of biological real talk, a crash course in hormones, songs about periods, and plenty of amazing advice for women and girls who haven't yet been given the chance to make friends with their menses. Her last run of sold out dates at the festival saw crowds of women, and men, waiting to talk to her afterwards, to share their excitement at just being able to talk openly about menstruation. *Ramona Magazine* has also developed a series of workshops called Period Witches, aimed at teenagers who want to learn how to get the most out of their menstrual cycle, in a cool, cute format. Meanwhile Rosie, a nationwide harm prevention initiative of the Dugdale Trust for Women & Girls, recently surveyed close to 1000 high school students, who said free menstrual products in schools was an urgent issue. The petition they are now circulating to demand this already has thousands of signatures, and those of us beyond school age have a clear indication that young people are aware that the menstrual taboo is an impediment to gender justice and they want it gone.

Working to end inequality is a massive social undertaking and the menstrual taboo cuts across it in so many ways. An organisation that really understands this is Share the Dignity, the Australian charity for women experiencing homelessness, poverty and those experiencing domestic violence through the distribution of menstrual products, and now, also, the funding of funerals for women who are victims of family violence. They estimate 85,000 women a year benefit from the work they have been doing since 2015, with around 3,000 volunteers across the country making it possible. In the UK, Hey Girls is dedicated to fighting period poverty by making sure that school-aged girls have access to the menstrual products they need, through donations, events and their public campaigns. They recently launched Pads 4 Dads, where the actor Michael Sheen joined the ranks of menstrual activists by helping draw attention to how many dads don't have the skills and information they need to be good supporters for the menstruating people in their families, especially daughters.

India has proven to be a powerful locus for menstrual activism with many having heard of the 'Pad Man', Arunachalam Muruganantham, the social entrepreneur who invented a low-cost machine to manufacture pads at a fraction of the price Indian women were faced with before. After discovering that his wife was managing her period with dirty rags in order to balance the household budget, due to the high cost of pads, he embarked on a long journey that eventually led him to worldwide fame. The Indian movies *Padman* and *Phullu* are both dramatised versions of his story, and the women who worked with him towards the goal of pads for everyone who needs them. The Oscar-winning documentary *Period. End of Sentence.* also tells the story of the pad machines from the perspective of a group of women in Hapur, India, who are learning to use them and in the process are becoming empowered to challenge the menstrual taboo in their country, at the same time as building their own economic independence. Alongside the film you can support The Pad Project, which aims to get these life-changing machines to communities of women who need them, by raising funds outside of India.

There's also momentum at the intersection of feminist art, culture, community and comedy. The Clams are Melbourne's premier feminist water ballerinas, merging synchronised swimming with period positivity and radical self-love. Their 2017 show 'Crimson Tide' combined cabaret with chlorine and brought the audience into the Melbourne Baths to see glamorous red-clad swimmers frolic with giant tampons to a selection of clever and cheeky tunes, including the genius addition of 'Crimson and Clover' (the Joan Jett version). They've since hosted body-positive pool parties and their follow-up show is dedicated to the full acceptance and celebration of women's body hair, the fabulously titled 'Grow Your Own Way', further highlighting the connection between menstrual wellbeing and overall body acceptance.

Hailing from the UK but touring around the world is the dark drama and magical horror of 'Dr Carnesky's Incredible Bleeding Woman', a show that 'reinvents menstrual rituals for a new era, drawing on the hidden power of a forgotten matriarchal past'. Drawing on Dr Marisa Carnesky's actual doctoral research in anthropology and her background as a self-described travelling showwoman, this deep dive into women and blood is funny, frightening and full of power, for the audience and the performers. It's another example of the way in which people are hungering for new narratives around menstruation that can reinvigorate our current perceptions of it, even as we uncover women's wisdom of the past. The work was also informed and supported by the formation of an activist arm, The Menstronauts, which you can find and join on Facebook, and learn more about ritual activism and your own menstrual cycle, as well as connect with groups around the world on the same journey. Importantly, both The Menstronauts and 'Dr Carnesky's Incredible Bleeding Woman' include trans women sharing their experiences of cycling, hormonal fluctuation and their deeper embodiment of womanhood through a physical and conceptual engagement with menstruation and menopause.

The UK also introduced the first trans man ever to appear in advertisements for menstrual products, when Kenny Jones featured in the 'I'm On' campaign for monthly period subscription service, Pink Parcel. He has spoken eloquently about how the menstrual taboo operated on him in different ways: 'It's something that's not talked about. I've never had a discussion with another trans man about periods and it's quite weird to think that considering it's a normal thing to go through at the end of the day.' In sharing such a valuable perspective, Jones not only normalises the reality that menstruation is very different for the men who experience it, but also highlights that openness and honesty are the keys to breaking down the idea that periods are somehow secret and shameful, for anyone. He put it beautifully when he said it's 'a very strange stigma that we shouldn't talk about it and I think that's a bad thing. It should be put in a positive light and say it's OK to talk about things. It's just a natural part of who we are, a normal body function'. Just a natural part of who we are.

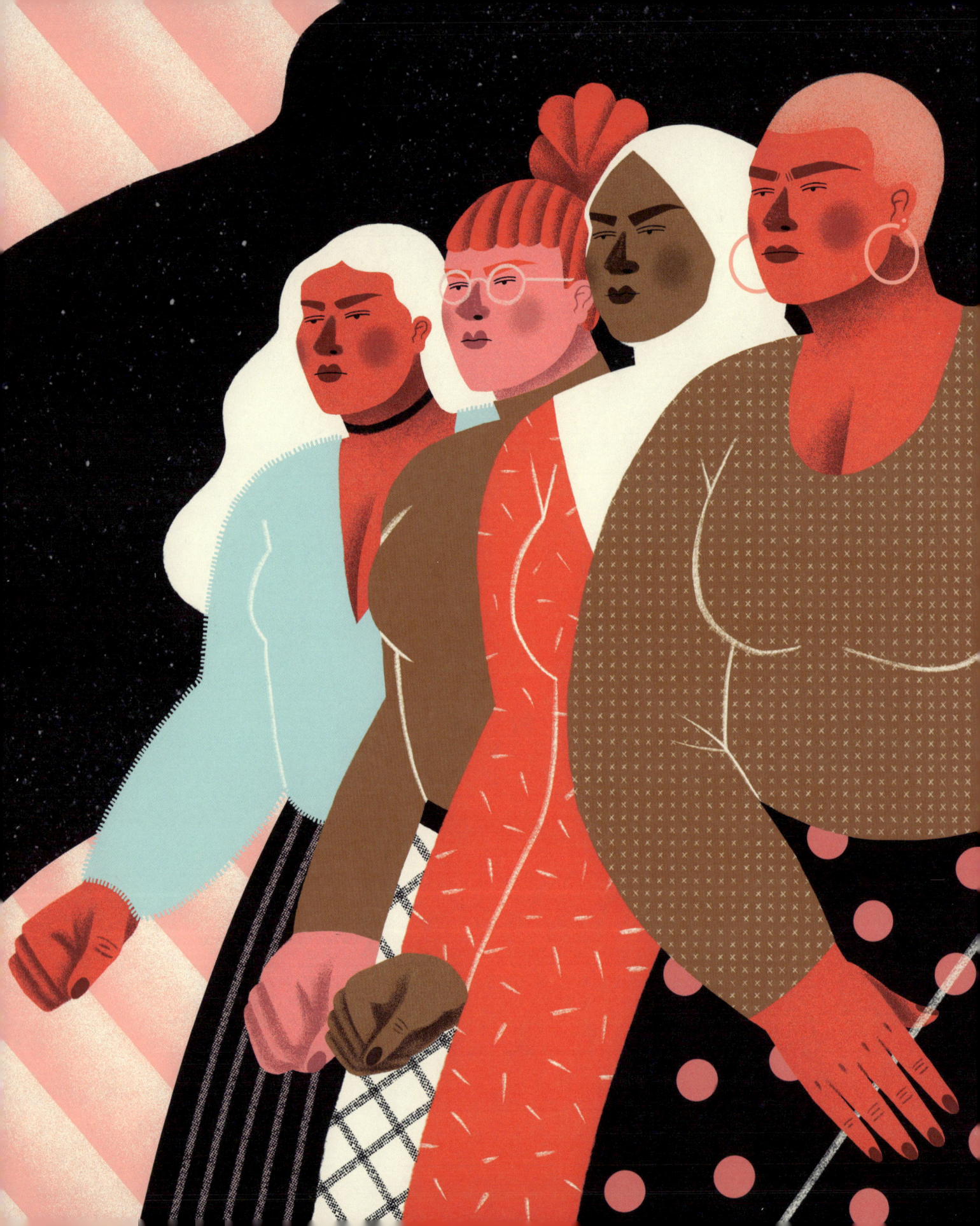

DISMANTLING THE MENSTRUAL TABOO

ABOUT BLOODY TIME

GIVEN THE PERVASIVENESS, IMPACT AND CONSEQUENCES of the menstrual taboo, is it really so radical to suggest that the menstrual taboo creates a lot of discord and difficulty, and nothing of real benefit, to women, girls, and the societies they build and inhabit? It costs us so much and gives us little in return. Why would we keep investing in it? Why wouldn't we divest our energy and refocus it elsewhere? It takes so much to keep upholding this archaic taboo; the waste, the harm, the compounded effects that reverberate throughout women's lives and place so much pressure on our families, our communities, not to mention our economic systems. But most important of all, when we know that a girl has more ambition, more confidence and more self-esteem before she starts menstruating than she does after, how can we go on like this?[i]

The dismantling of an unproductive and unhelpful menstrual taboo starts with a vision of how things can be otherwise. One of our respondents put it beautifully:

> *I dream of a world where menstruation is normalised and honoured for the miraculous process it is and respected for its biological and cultural challenges.*

This woman's dream is not romantic or unachievable. But we do have to be able to creatively place ourselves in a different menstrual reality.

Imagine.

A girl is in her bathroom at home and she notices something different. It's red. Or is it brown? It's on her underpants. She hasn't seen it before. Her heart starts thumping and she feels ... scared? Excited? Amazed? Surprised? Yes. She calls out to her parents, who come to the door and ask if she's okay. 'I am,' she says. 'I think I've got my period.' It's here. She was prepared for this, and now, after much anticipation, it is really happening. There are happy tears, on both sides of the door. Overwhelming feelings! Some fear of the unknown? Of course! A little worry and confusion too, but the preparation kicks in, with a sense of power. A flurry of activity: grabbing supplies, hugs, lots of hugs, planning tonight's dinner, thinking about gifts, congratulations, reassurance, calling aunties, grandmas, cousins, who will want to celebrate. She grasps the sense of occasion. She knows that what is happening to her is normal and natural, but also important and momentous. She is a little apprehensive about her life changing now, but she is also proud, excited and can't wait to tell her friends.

Her home is like many others, with parents teaching their children with confidence and comfort about the practicalities of self-care and managing periods. School is also a safe and supportive space, free of judgment and stigma, not least of all because students and teachers have benefited hugely from the national educational framework to implement menstrual wellbeing: concept and practice, into the school curriculum. She grows up to work in environments with modern, progressive attitudes towards women and their periods, many having menstrual policies in place to ensure that all workers are supported to be their most productive, creative and whole selves. Women are likewise comfortable being open and honest in their relationships and approach to sex, knowing their bodies as strong, powerful sites of pleasure, desire and possibility. Most importantly, women and girls know that their bodies are their own, and they expect everybody, in every context, to respect this fact. No exceptions, no compromise: women own themselves.

The societal respect for women's bodies extends to the healthcare system, where all Australian women and girls are provided with holistic, attentive and respectful treatment, underpinned by the acceptance of menstrual wellbeing as a key factor in overall health and quality of life. Contraception and conception are assisted ably, with the informed consent and personal agency of every woman respected and safeguarded. For women who experience menstrual dysfunction, and menstruation related illness, diagnosis is swift and clear, with appropriate treatments (including advice about lifestyle, medication, physical therapy and surgery) offered promptly, safely and effectively, giving women real choices while alleviating pain and distress. Advances in scientific knowledge, due to adequate and fair funding, flow through to the frontlines rapidly, and now guarantee that no Australian woman will be ignored or disbelieved again, when reporting her extreme pain or debilitating periods to a medical professional. The national framework to introduce menstrual wellbeing into the medical community and healthcare curriculum has already changed industry practice, and better care for menopausal and peri-menopausal women has also been assured, improving the lives of millions of Australians, across generations.

We have changed the culture to one that values menstruation for the extraordinary process that it is, and so values women accordingly, with men also playing a critical role in this shift. Thanks to the hard work, persistence and courage of women and girls, menstrual educators, policymakers, legislators, employers, teachers, doctors, unionists, scientists, academics, artists, journalists, public servants and an active and engaged citizenry, the menstrual taboo has been relegated to history, where it belongs.

This vision of menstrual wellbeing will require change, imaginative ideas for action, national policy, political will, resources and money, persistence, bravery and most important of all, collaboration.

Historians have built careers on trying to pinpoint the exact moment a revolution begins. In some cases, to tell a cautionary tale, to prevent it ever happening again and breaching the peace with the kind of upheaval that reinvents societies and changes the course of history. Other times, it is because they are looking for that blend of social and political forces, that in some combination gives rise to a movement for change that, from a certain moment, proceeds with ineluctable and unstoppable force. In our case, such a moment will never be divined. Not only because menstruation is older than the menstrual taboo, but because the energy that drives our revolution forward now is so diffuse, so varied, so complex, and so embedded in so many different cultures around the world and across time, that a starting point does not exist. There hasn't always, or in every culture, been negativity and hostility towards menstruation, but right now it is measurable in most.

Change is in motion: a menstrual revolution is happening, and we have the chance to build the kind of infrastructure that will see it liberate all women and girls from the injuries of the menstrual taboo, and make the whole of society healthier, happier and more harmonious.

The removal of GST from menstrual products is to be applauded, and it represents an agreement that it was wrong to tax these items when it began in 2000. It was wrong to tax them then, and it was wrong every year since. In the meantime, millions of Australian women, over two decades, have contributed taxation revenue in the order of nearly half a billion dollars by paying GST on tampons and pads. There has been a massive over collection of tax, specifically from one group of Australian taxpayers: women.

There is a strong argument to be made for retrospective redress. Given the centrality of menstrual wellbeing to the overall health and wellbeing of women, it makes huge sense that a significant allocation of funds; equal to or comparable in size to this wrongly collected tax, should be reinvested back into women's health, specifically into areas which will build positive menstrual and menopausal culture.

If you think that sounds ambitious and far-reaching, we agree. What we are proposing is a cultural, institutional and public health response that is absolutely appropriate in scale to an issue that affects over half the population: changes in legislation, in education, in health care, in our workplaces, and across our broader culture. The research is so clear – we consider it a kind of moral mandate to proceed with optimism, confidence and hope that with the following five key areas addressed, we will start to see significant and powerful change inside of a generation.

1. Menstrual policy as standard practice in all Australian workplaces

All Australian workplaces operate within the parameters of legislation and compliance to national, state and local regulatory bodies. They also have their own suite of policies relating to the work environment, behaviour and standards. For example, a firm may have a social media policy, a policy around reporting accidents, and policies regarding dress standards or mobile phone use at work.

A menstrual policy would take its place alongside these other measures for promoting consistency, clarity and a safe, constructive working environment for employees and employers alike. A good start is with the Menstrual and Menopause Wellbeing Policy developed by the Victorian Women's Trust (see Appendix Four). The instrument for ensuring that menstrual policies are incorporated as standard practice will be a series of criteria to be met by participating organisations, with some type of financial incentive. This would ensure that uptake of the menstrual policies across the board would be swift and widespread.

For decades, women have agitated for equal rights in workplaces, around issues like pay equity, parental leave, the eradication of sexual harassment and representation of women on boards. These are all pressing concerns underpinning the advancement of women in workplaces that have been fashioned historically by men, without adapting or accommodating the needs of women as they have increasingly formed a significant part of the paid workforce. Introducing menstrual policies into workplaces is the next logical step in bringing about truly women-positive spaces in which every employee has the chance to reach their full productive potential. Achieving this through formal, legislative measures, within a national framework that provides support, assistance and templates for change, will result in better workplaces for women, their colleagues and their employers.

Our research painted such a clear picture of workplaces being a site of major anxiety and disconnection for women as they balance the demands of their job with the needs of their body and their selves around menstruation and menopause. The simple and decent act of consulting with employees to form an official menstrual policy for a workplace is a decision that many employers can make executively, before seeing the obvious benefits. As a driver of broader social change, we'd like to see visionary employers take up the challenge to lead the way in terms of establishing menstrual policies at work, to bring Australia forward into the 21st century, where our economy is driven by men and women who can lay claim to building truly modern and equal workplaces.

> *I would love to speak about it without whispering. My employer is really good, but I would like other employees to be more open. I'm tired of the shameful silence and hiding my pads.*

> *My pain and nausea is really bad for at least the first day or two every menstruation, but period pain is not taken seriously where I work and I'm expected to just deal with it. I can't pay for a doctor's appointment to get a certificate every time I go home early just because my ovaries hate me. It's really tough and comes around with alarming regularity.*

> *When I worked in hospitality as a casual there was no way I could have taken time off for feeling crummy when I had my period. Even when I was exhausted from being up all night in pain I just had to suck it up and fight my need to sit or slow down. No work, no pay and*

absolutely no room for discussion. It was all about the bottom line. In my current workplace a menstrual policy was introduced a couple of years ago after conversations about periods generally and our own needs in particular.

Partly through these conversations and partly through the menstrual policy I felt a real sense of relief and support. I felt relieved that now I don't have to pretend I am fine when I'm not and can be honest about what I am feeling. I feel supported because this part of me is heard and seen and validated. It wasn't until we had the Menstrual Policy that I realised how much effort it had taken to ignore my menstrual symptoms previously or at least pretend they weren't happening. These might variously be a headache, extreme tiredness, depression, pain or a combination of them.

Now having the option to work from home on my first day has made an amazing difference. I can make myself comfortable with a hot water bottle on my belly, I can avoid spending an hour and a half on my feet commuting and I can still get my work done. One of my colleagues said recently that she realised that, 'understanding your cycle is a feminist act' and I really think that's true. Also, I think that the conversation has created a more compassionate atmosphere at work. We feel more able to look after ourselves and our wellbeing is respected both for its own sake and also for the overall productivity of our workplace.

2. A new public health standard regarding menstrual wellbeing to be incorporated into our health care system

Public health is a central pillar of our society, representing a practical application of the value placed on the wellbeing of individuals and of the community as a whole. The parameters of public health are prevention, risk mitigation, diagnosis, alleviation of symptoms and cure, as well as the ethical considerations involved in these. Public health authorities plan and resource the health care of the overall population, subgroups within the community and the specific needs of individuals, at least to the capacity of resources and appreciation of need.

Central to the successful operation of public health programs are the standards that provide guidelines for delivery. These standards emerge through identification of need, discussion and debate, and reflect a commitment to monitoring, improving and guaranteeing service delivery outcomes. For instance, there are standards that govern birthing and neo-natal care, cancer screening, diagnosis and treatment, diabetes management and prevention, failure to thrive in children, eye and ear health, emergency triage, pap smears and breast screens and end of life care. These are just a few examples. Surely it makes sense to see menstrual wellbeing added to this list; from menarche to menopause, women and girls should be able to access the very best support and treatment available regarding their menstrual health.

Of course, new standards come into existence regularly, and all are scrutinised, changed and improved as science and practical considerations evolve. Sometimes standards even slip. One thing is certain though and that is that standards in public health will always be evolving and adapting, hopefully in response to new developments and changing need. Nevertheless, the mission of public health, and its standards, is to conceptualise, plan and deliver health benefits to the whole community.

In the dynamic and diverse realm of public health resourcing, delivery and promotion, it is inconceivable that there currently exists nothing relating to menstrual health and no standard defining menstrual wellbeing, across our entire healthcare system. How can it be that this physical process that is so critical to a woman's life, her wellbeing and her health, is largely ignored by the public health system? When menstruation is only approached and understood under the rubric of reproductive and sexual health, women will continue to be short changed by our medical system.

Women have suffered too long with a public health system lacking any standards or guidance for menstrual wellbeing, for both practitioners and patients. When the average woman in Australia spends six to seven years of her life menstruating and nearly 40 years altogether cycling, we need a responsive and sophisticated approach to this field of women's health. In her lifetime, she is likely to deal with pain, fatigue, mood fluctuations, cycle-related anxiety, fertility issues, extremes of menstrual flow, headaches, digestive discomfort and very often dismissiveness or delayed diagnosis when engaging health professionals for problems pertaining to her cycle, including during peri-menopause and menopause.

> *I wish I had known much earlier that periods don't have to be painful – something that you just have to put up with – that you can seek help, make dietary adjustments, use exercise techniques and natural therapies, and use contraceptive methods other than the Pill.*

> *We can help ourselves so much by listening to our intuition, to our bodies, possibly changing our diets, our habits and patterns, using herbs and other natural non-invasive remedies to minimise difficult symptoms. We now have a wealth of information to help us make positive decisions about what is best for us as individuals. We need to accept that we are growing older with equanimity, at the very least, if not excitement!*

3. National health education and promotion programs focused on menstrual wellbeing

Menstrual wellbeing needs to be carefully and comprehensively defined in consultation with experts, and then embedded at all levels of health care with an amply resourced education program for healthcare professionals and the industry, to be accompanied by an ongoing health promotion campaign for the general public. This level of investment will bring about improved health for all women, which impacts the whole of society in measurable and positive ways. Much like earlier public health campaigns in Australia, including our responses to reduce drink-driving, skin cancer, and addressing the HIV/AIDS crisis, this program to introduce menstrual wellbeing to medical professionals and all the women in their care, will be world's best practice and observed for years to come as the gold standard in interventionist progressive public health.

An improved public health response around menstrual wellbeing can be triggered immediately through the establishment of a national task force, through which guidelines can be developed and incorporated within 36 months, to become a national standard of care and treatment for women and girls, from menarche through to menopause and beyond.

The need to build and support a positive menstrual culture for girls and women throughout their lives, for parents and schools, and for the whole community is indisputable. We need to see an official fund to be endowed at the national level in order to work with the best menstrual educators and relevant agencies to develop and deliver this material across the country. This would allow accredited providers to apply for funding from a central body, to produce the best resources and tools for making this change in Australian society. This kind of model can realistically be built within the next five years, which would see generational change begin almost immediately, towards the concept of menstrual wellbeing becoming an accepted part of our culture, improving the lives of girls and women immeasurably.

Men should not be apprehensive about periods. They should be educated and comfortable about the function of menstruation, instead of being disgusted and avoiding any discussion about it. Start educating boys about menstruation. They are taught at a young age by macho apes to crack jokes about menstruation, and to demean and disregard women because of this natural process. Too many men will, if you disagree with them, say, 'What, are you on the rag or somethin'?!' What a great way for men to belittle women.

Teaching young women about the sacred nature of menstruation, birth and female community seems to me to be crucial for connecting us to female power, and for overturning negative attitudes about menstruation, body image and self-worth.

Feeling seriously uninformed about my pending menopause, and rather frightened by the prospect, I just went to a weekend workshop about it. I'm so glad I did! It was so not the doom and gloom and focus on symptoms that I'd found on the internet. We learnt about the self-care that will make a big difference, and what I need to be doing right now. Just talking with other women for a whole weekend was exhilarating. I feel empowered to start looking after myself better with chiropractic for some chronic issues, yoga, cutting out sugar and less stress, just for a start. I'm really excited now about the prospect of menopause and what my life can be in this next important phase.

It is a wonderful experience that has been so vilified and feared by patriarchal society. Each woman honouring her own body and its natural rhythms is going to heal it for us all.

When I was a teenager I was so terribly embarrassed if anyone knew I had my period. Now it has become a common topic of conversation amongst my friends and is a genuine connection between us.

I'm part of an online women's forum and we have a thread talking about our menstruation experiences. From practical tips to everyone's openness and honesty it's been a really supportive and beneficial group.

4. The provision of menstrual products as standard practice, alongside other amenities like toilet paper and soap

Public toilets are a significant public amenity. They exist because we agree, as a society, to fund the costs of meeting the needs of our citizenry to access amenities as a basic human right. In a public toilet, we reasonably expect to find toilet paper and soap, sometimes paper towel or a hand dryer, and usually doors that lock and maybe even a mirror. These represent amenity and convenience, but they also speak to the idea that we think people have the right to go to the toilet, to relieve themselves and not be caught in public without access to the facilities we need for comfort and cleanliness. Does it not make sense then, that alongside toilet paper and soap, public toilets would also provide products that are routinely required by roughly half the population? We know that women and girls sometimes face difficult situations around managing their periods, with most of us having been caught without the supplies we need to deal with unexpected arrivals. The cost of adding these supplies to the current roster of what is considered essential in a public bathroom would constitute a small difference to the overall budget of providers. Nonetheless it would make a huge difference to the lives of women and girls, whether disadvantaged or just caught out, as well as send a message that dignifies and normalises their experience. We should consider supplying these items for free, even if it means that the Commonwealth subsidises local government (who would be largely responsible for implementation) with annual grants to cover the cost. Balancing the benefits to women and girls against the expected costs makes it clear that the former would be significant while the latter almost negligible.

In the mid-1980s, a woman had her period arrive unexpectedly while flying from Brisbane to Melbourne. She asked the hostess if they carried any sorts of pads. No was the reply. But the hostess did manage to find some from another hostess. The woman wrote to the airline suggesting it would be a good policy for the airline to have supplies on board to benefit women. No response was forthcoming (personal communication with staff at the VWT).

This question of providing menstrual products as standard practice should not be limited to toilets. Now that we've thoroughly interrogated the menstrual taboo it's time to look at the ways in which it has stopped us from making sensible decisions around public amenity and access to facilities of convenience.

5. Taxation on menstrual products be deemed off limits in any future negotiations on budget repair or boosting taxation revenue

Through the decades-long dedication and hard work of activists and campaigners an historic wrong has been overturned and the so-called 'tampon tax' removed. What is now required is an ironclad commitment, agreed on by the major parties, that any taxation on menstrual products will be completely off limits going forward, so that future generations of women and girls will not face the same situation again. This is, in many respects, the most straightforward and easily attainable of our goals. It simply asks that future legislators and elected representatives refrain from using menstrual products as a political football, in order to score points for, or against, certain constituencies.

In conclusion

Our research and writing for this publication were a gender and social-justice initiative funded by the Victorian Women's Trust and The Dugdale Trust for Women & Girls, with a special focus on the stated goal of the latter: meaningful harm prevention for girls and women, especially as it pertains to menstruation and menopause. As the project evolved, and more and more women shared their experiences, the full extent of this harm became apparent, and what also became clear was the near total inadequacy of existing structures to mitigate and improve it. Despite the dedicated work of menstrual educators and activists in this space for decades, it became obvious that large-scale social change would be required to not only address the pervasiveness and harmfulness of the menstrual taboo, but to conceive of a new way: to liberate women and girls and allow them the right to a positive relationship with their menstrual cycle.

> *I'm a midwife and I recently started at a new workplace. I was surprised and delighted to find packets of pads and tampons open on the bench in the staff toilets. Our midwifery unit is in a really busy city women's hospital and to have this taken care of feels very supportive, matter-of-fact and just sensible really. The last thing any of us need in the middle of a shift is to be fussing about searching for a tampon in the storeroom or our locker when it can even be a stretch finding time to go to the toilet. Thank you, administrators!*

The changes we propose are ambitious and comprehensive, but they are also logical and achievable. As we move closer to achieving gender equality we will need to keep the pressure on governments to formulate policy and legislation that builds infrastructure for change, rather than waiting for that change to miraculously occur.

Equity is not inevitable but rather the result of relentless dedication and commitment on the part of change agents in the community – not only organisers, campaigners and activists but ordinary people working together to make our society better for everyone. We want to see more respect and understanding for menstruating (and menopausal) women and girls in every sphere of their lives, and that means we take our message everywhere; to governments and schools, to universities and hospitals, courtrooms and workplaces, to sporting clubs and unions.

This menstrual revolution, perhaps ironically, won't be bloody. Like all progressive social movements, it asks us to call on our better natures to see the truth of a former injustice, and it comes together as our way of getting to a future where we can all be liberated.

The revolution might have originated in women passing down their truths over generations but now we know how much everyone can gain from understanding menstrual wellbeing. The knowledge underpinning this revolution comes from women, but it seeks to benefit everybody. The perpetuation of the menstrual taboo stultifies relationships between women and men, boys and girls, and in fact has a deleterious effect on all people and our civic culture. It demeans and subordinates women by sabotaging their self-confidence, restricting their bodily autonomy, and it actively harms the prospects for genuine equality and equity. Dismantling the taboo and replacing it with a truly positive menstrual culture not only liberates women and girls but will be a powerful contributor and precursor to what so many Australians want: a more just and equitable world for all.

The taboo subordinates women, but, not for the first time, women are pushing back. We know the power of rejecting the limits placed on us. We embrace the potential of being insubordinate. We are seeking nothing less than a demolition of the menstrual taboo. We can make this happen, and in fact replace it with a positive, powerful concept of menstrual wellbeing, that is experienced across our society in meaningful connections between women, girls and their communities.

ABOUT BLOODY TIME

> *My period was the first thing that felt truly mine, the beginning of my autonomy as a young woman. The beginning of my rising, my rebellion, my striving for freedom and safety.*

Recalling our earlier introduction of Bex Baxter and her persuasive TED Talk on introducing a menstrual policy to her organisation, we wanted to share a particular lesson she took with her. Recounting her experience, she described how she went home and 'felt a very strange and unfamiliar sensation: "I'm allowed to be here and look after myself" … I realised that the shame wasn't there … and I called it 'the permission field'. It's a culture of trust that relieves the stress, anxiety and shame of taking menstrual leave. We realised that the fear of these judgments was often crippling, and actually increased the suffering brought on by our periods'. This notion of a 'permission field' is arresting and powerful – the very idea that the menstrual shame, anxiety and physical effects can be alleviated when a culture of mutual trust is established; when society reflects the fact that every woman has the right to care for herself, across her cycle and throughout the stages of her life, we will elevate and confirm the agency of all women.

The idea of a 'permission field' can be illuminating and instructive on a larger scale too. Baxter describes the menstrual policy of her workplace as vital in recognising the permission she now had to look after herself; but it also gave her permission to see menstruation as a collective experience for women and a field in which she might agitate for change. In leveraging her experience as motivation to speak about menstrual policies at work, she shared their positive impact on her and her workplace and advocated for wider social and institutional change. When women see they have permission to regard menstruation with emotions other than shame and anxiety, and unite around these deeply shared experiences, so will their collective lateral power increase. When the permission field extends to women collectively, the pace and force of social change gathers to become much greater than the significance of one woman looking after herself. Then you have a revolution.

> *My period is a check in, a time to stop and ask, what do I need in this moment? How can I support myself? With four young kids I don't get to do that often but I'm definitely more gentle with myself when I bleed.*

> *I was given a Mood Diary for my birthday when I was 22. It was beautiful, and I loved spending quiet time with it reflecting and writing. Over time it really helped me to appreciate my periods and cyclic changes, and this became a powerful self-awareness to live my life by.*

> *Learning to respect and work with my cycle rather than pushing myself through it has been one of the tools that has helped me heal from depression. I'm so happy that my feelings toward having periods have changed, that I learned to use the energy of menstruation to go deep within and that I started giving myself permission to rest.*

When the whole of society sees women's bodies as dynamic, deserving of respect, and valuable in their own right, we will transform the world we live in. This is absolutely crucial to the broader project of achieving full gender equality. Contributing to that process; by helping girls and women to see their bodies as powerful and full of potential; is open to all of us. Breaking the deadlocks of shame, anxiety and fear, by connecting menstruation to vitality, health, integrity and dignity: this is what we mean when we talk about revolutionising menstrual culture.

The revolution has already begun and it's about bloody time.

Acknowledgements

The Victorian Women's Trust (VWT Ltd) and its harm prevention entity, The Dugdale Trust for Women & Girls (DTWG), would like to credit and acknowledge the many people who have assisted the realisation of this important project initiative.

Phase One: October 2013 – September 2015

Project initiation, data collection and report compilation

Project Advisory Group: Jane Bennett, Jane Hardwick Collings, Katherine Cunningham, Duré Dara OAM and Bindy (Belinda) Gross

Donor support: We thank our generous and inaugural donor, Bindy Gross, for enabling us to proceed to first stage of the project. We thank our wonderful donors, regular and occasional, for supporting our work and enabling us to bring initiatives such as *About Bloody Time* to fruition. We also thank everyone who enthusiastically climbed on board and supported our recent Pozible campaign. Quite simply, we couldn't have done this without you all.

VWT/DTWG staff: Mary Crooks AO (Project Director), Lara Owen (Project Leader), Adrienne Bogard (Project Officer), Ally Oliver-Perham (Design and Communications), Wilfredo Zelada (Financial Management)

Initial design and logistics for the state-wide discussion groups: Kat Romei and Adrienne Bogard

Discussion group hosts and volunteer convenors: Lucy Armstrong, Jo Clifford, Samantha Fernandez, Monica Francia, Melissa Gonella, Naina Knoess, Janoel Liddy, Denise Martin, Katy Meltzer, Ingrid Petterson, Ari Rutman, Elly Scrine, Sharon Syman Etzion, Bec Vandyke and Melinda Whyman

Teachers and school staff involved in the Secondary School Conversation Groups: Lyn Farrow, Karen Glanc, Lesley Milne, Briony O'Keefe and Pauline Rice

External support: Lydia Brown, Deanne Carson, Gedis Grudzinskas, Gavin Jack, Monique Jansonius, Dr Sharon Maloney, Dr Christiane Northrup, Alexandra Pope, Kat Riach, Imelda Roche, Kate Seear, Yolanda Vega and Paul Zappa

Volunteers and interns: Emma Buckley Lennox, Rachel Etzion, Lucy Fahey, Melissa Gonella, Ruby Hedigan-Dattner, Mary Keely, Janoel Liddy, Federica Marzari, Madeline McGlade and Pat Stragalinos

Research Report lodged September 2015: Lara Owen and Adrienne Bogard

Independent Assessment of Research Report: Dr Louise Keogh, Associate Professor School of Population and Global Health, The University of Melbourne

Phase Two: October 2015 – March 2019
Data analysis – development and production of full manuscript for publication

Project Advisory Group: Project Advisory Group: Jane Bennett, Jane Hardwick Collings, Katherine Cunningham, Bindy Gross (resigned 2017) and Duré Dara OAM

Core writing team: Karen Pickering and Jane Bennett

Project Director: Mary Crooks AO

Research Analyst: Nicole Isles

Medical Terminology and references: Dr Danielle Arbena

External support: Jen Hargrave and Keran Howe (Women's Disability Victoria), Dr Jane Mallick, Angela Hywood and Emily Maguire

Volunteers and Interns: Pam Carty-Salmon and Denise Keighery (assimilation of the qualitative data and reference materials) and Bronwyn Dwyer (research materials and references)

VWT/DTWG staff: Casimira Melican and Maria Chetcuti for reviews of draft manuscript and Wilfredo Zelada for financial management and project support. All who participated at our 7 August 2018 review workshop – Gillian Barnes, Sophie Bliss, Alice Chambers, Maria Chetcuti, Maddy Crehan, Duré Dara OAM, Esther Davies-Brown, Nikky Friedman, Hilary Irwin, Casimira Melican, Ally Oliver-Perham and Wilfredo Zelada. Finally, Claire Duffy and Casimira Melican for editing the manuscript.

The VWT Board: led by Alana Johnson (Chair), for their support and patience as a complex and challenging project came to fruition.

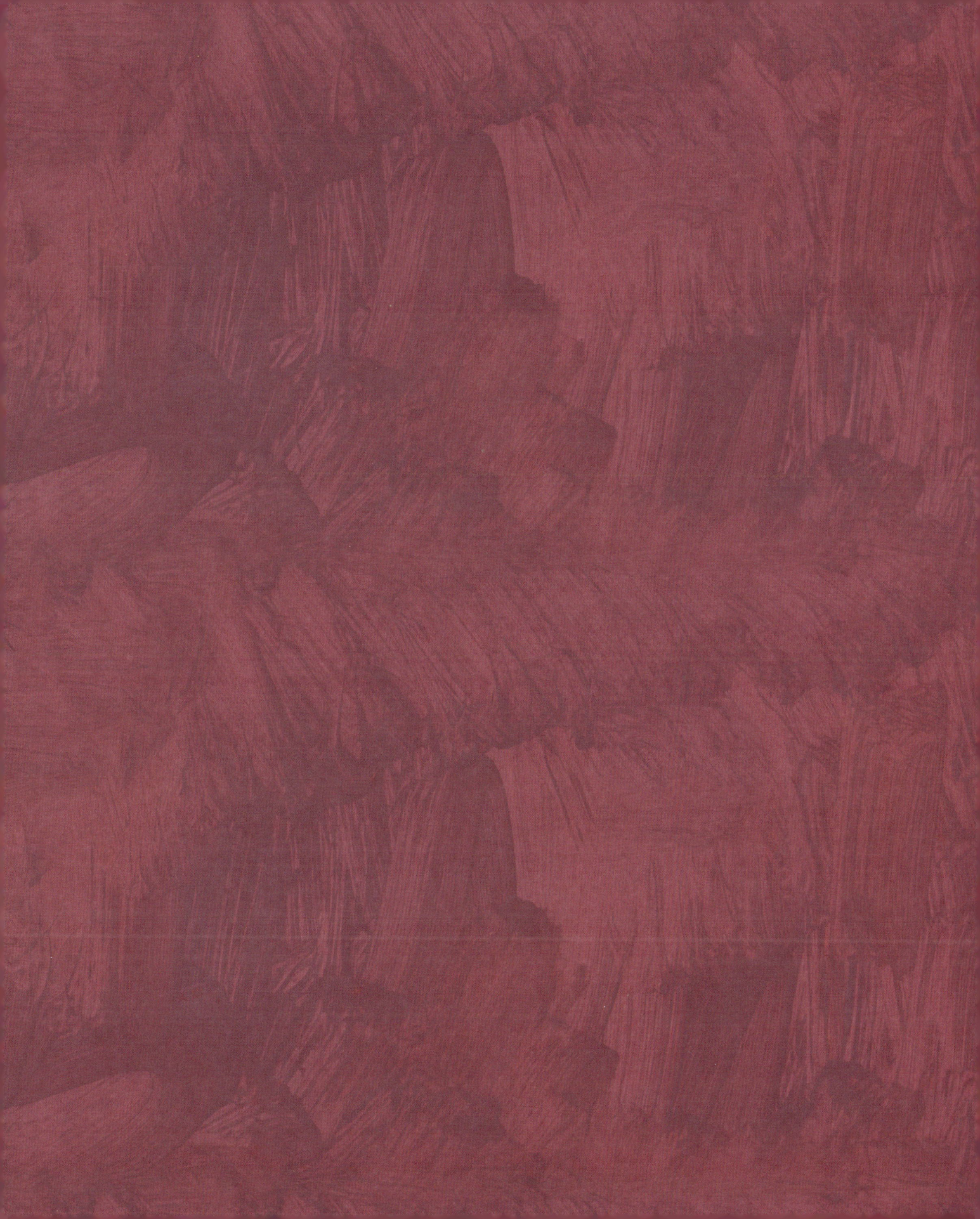

Appendix One: Methodology

The Dugdale Trust for Women and Girls (Victorian Women's Trust as trustee) committed to The Waratah Project, in December 2012. The aim was to explore women's and girls' experience of menarche, menstruation and menopause and develop a landmark narrative that could inform progressive change for positive menstruation and the wellbeing of women and girls.

The project methodology consisted of literature review, online survey and kitchen table discussion groups.

The literature review

An extensive review of existing research was made, across a range of academic disciplines, as well as those by corporations and women's organisations, with particular attention paid to research that questioned women directly. In addition, a range of experts in related fields were interviewed.

The questionnaire survey

Questionnaires were created for age groups:

- girls 12-18
- women 19-30
- women 31-45
- and two for women 46 plus
  - one for those who still menstruated and
  - one for those who had transitioned through menopause.

The questionnaires were slightly different for each age group, depending on stage of fertile life and life generally, and took into consideration: menarche status, use of ovulation and/or menstruation supressing drugs, school and work, pregnancy, menopause and aging. The questionnaires in the second active period of gathering responses in 2016 included a question asking whether a

APPENDIX ONE

woman identified as having a disability, and if she did, whether this impacted on her menstrual or menopausal experience.

All the surveys had a mix of responses where respondents could answer multiple-choice questions and write comments of any length.

The total number of respondents was 3460, 342 of whom attended discussion groups as well. The age breakdown was: 247 girls 12 to 18 years old, 781 young women 19 to 30 years old, 1197 women 31 to 45 and 1235 women 46 years old and over. Of the latter a greater number were post-menopausal, with the oldest respondent being 80 years old.

Of the women and girls who responded to the survey online 51% were from Australia, 30% from the United States, 7% from Canada and 4% from the United Kingdom. The remaining 8% were from a further 51 countries, including Argentina, Austria, Belarus, Belgium, Brazil, Bulgaria, Costa Rica, Croatia, Curacao, Cyprus, Denmark, Ecuador, Estonia, Finland, France, Georgia, Germany, Greece, Guatemala, Hong Kong, India, Ireland, Israel, Italy, Japan, Kenya, Malaysia, Malta, Mexico, The Netherlands, New Zealand, Norway, Pakistan, Peru, Portugal, Romania, Russia, Singapore, Slovenia, South Africa, South Korea, Spain, Sweden, Switzerland, Thailand, Timor-Leste, Trinidad and Tobago, Tunisia, Turkey, United Arab Emirates and Uruguay.

The survey process meant that respondents self-selected. As such there are no claims made of the results being representative or statistically significant. This important qualification aside, the survey results provide unique and rich insight into the experience of menarche, menstruation and menopause.

The sample was complex and diverse, however it was beyond the scope of the research to determine the race, ethnicity, physical capability and sexuality of every respondent. That said, many of the responses reference these identity markers and wherever possible we include them to give a broader picture of women's experience. In some ideal future there will be specialised studies and resources on menstruation and menopause that focus primarily on the contemporary experience of diverse people.

Kitchen table conversations

To compliment the survey questionnaire, the Victorian Women's Trust model of 'kitchen table' conversations groups was adopted. Twenty-two discussion groups were held across urban and rural Victoria between April and November 2014, at these locations: Armidale, Belgrave, Briar Hill, Castlemaine, Caulfield, Drouin, Eltham, Fitzroy, Geelong, Hawthorn and Hawthorn East, Launching Place, Melbourne CBD, Preston and Wangaratta. Women were asked to share their experiences and views, as well as fill in the questionnaire relevant to them.

In the conversation groups in schools, girls were asked for their views, but not to share their personal experiences, unless they freely volunteered to do so.

No names or identifying details were asked for and participants gave permission for their responses to be collected for survey purposes.

All discussion groups were audio recorded and transcribed for research and writing purposes.

Data analysis

Quantitative data were analysed in the quarter January to March 2017 by Nicole Isles, Master of Public Health candidate at the Melbourne School of Population and Global Health at Melbourne University, using Stata 14.2 software.

Appendix Two: Qualitative Data

Reflecting on first periods

Girls 12-15

Fine, I knew I was going through a natural thing • Terrified for a while, now I'm 98% fine with it • really hard to tell people, especially my mum • really emotional and moody towards everyone • very sad because I wanted to be able to swim all the time • like jumping into the unknown • relieved because my friends had theirs • pretty shit, to be honest • I was surprised and annoyed because I was playing murder in the dark and had to stop • like my childhood was over • I thought it was tomato sauce because I had fish and chips beforehand • I was scared and started crying • fine as my best friend had already told me about it • I didn't know if my friends had it or not so I felt alone • I didn't know what was going on • horrible pain • very worried for two reasons. 1. I didn't want my friends finding out. 2. I didn't want to grow up and be constantly scared I was on my period • trapped, like, "oh so this is what I'm going to have for a lot of my life" • I was a bit happy because a lot of other people in my class had got theirs and also coz if anyone had any trouble I could say "Oh yeah, I did this" • very surprised and kinda freaked out • I thought I'd never get it so I was relieved I was able to have children • I didn't know you could just get it without peeing so I was sort of confused • frightened, I didn't tell anybody • so excited to have come to a new stage of my life • I felt very weird and wouldn't move or anything, I just sat and did nothing • the pads were so uncomfy! • I felt nervous, a bit worried and a tiny bit more grown up • wow! I guess I'm a lady now • my friend was the one that noticed it was on my jeans. I didn't really care. I just cleaned up and went along with my day • worried about all the blood and laundry and intense cramping •

Girls 16-18

Menstruation was a topic of fascination and I was really excited to experience it for myself • I remember coming home and making myself a celebration milkshake but not telling my younger sister why • I felt sick and had a lot of cramps the night before • nervous and grossed out •

I dreaded the day I first got my period, I was terrified of growing up. I participate quite heavily in sport and was extremely anti-tampon, so I was worried about how it would affect my performance • I thought periods were disgusting and never talked about them with my friends • quite scared to tell my mum and ask her for help • I felt too young • excited! I was finally a woman woohoo! • really sad, really annoyed, like this was a great burden I'd have to deal with for the rest of my life • defined me as a woman, not a girl • it freaked me out that my body was ready for children at thirteen • relieved as I was one of the last few in my class • my parents were overseas and my older brothers were looking after me. It was really awkward • happy, surprised, relieved I got it at home • I had no idea what to do and was too scared to ask for help • sort of excited, like I was turning into a woman • I had such bad cramps and I was so embarrassed in front of my grade six class on camp that I was just puking and crying • I was kind of excited but I was also scared about how to tell mum • I was almost proud • I was worried it was internal bleeding • at first I thought I'd cut myself down there. Mum explained it was my period • I was scared and for a few months I hid it and tried to deal with it by myself • whatever. It didn't bother me •

Young women 19-30

I messaged my best friend explaining the colour and texture. She said it sounded like my period and to speak to my mum • Mum explained how to use a pad and was very gentle about the whole process • I saw the blood and panicked • I was at my dad's house and felt weird telling him thinking what would he know? • I felt totally mortified by the proof that I had a vagina • I immediately taught myself how to use tampons because the 6th grade pool party was coming up • I was shell shocked that it had actually happened. It took a while to get the hang of it • I would have felt more prepared if I wasn't so afraid • I knew the logistics, but it was still a bizarre thing to experience for the first time. I was not prepared for how my body felt • I was at a friend's house and was too embarrassed to ask for a pad • it took me the best part of that day to tell my mother • I thought I was having uncontrollable diarrhoea for days before I admitted to my mum what was happening • nobody told me about them, I was nine and really pissed because I was at school • Mum found my undies and told me • I thought I hadn't wiped my bum properly after pooing and vowed to do a better job going forward • I was a tomboy and Mum told me when it happened I had to wear skirts • I wasn't prepared for the pain or how much blood • Mum never had the talk with me • I didn't tell my mum for two days because I didn't know what she would say. I felt ashamed that I had started my period at such a young age as I had already developed C-cup breasts and a male teacher a few weeks before had told my mother that I needed high neck swimmers because I 'had the body of a woman' and I apparently 'knew it' at ten years old • I saw the blood on my undies and I burst into tears from shock • I thought I'd spilt my Ribena! • I thought I was internally bleeding and maybe needed to go to the hospital • only my dad was at home, he called a female family friend to come and help me out • I simply slapped on a pad and went about my business • I had been looking forward to it since I grew 'niplets' • I cried by myself in the toilet because I knew I could be a mother now but had no idea how to be a mother and that scared me (I wasn't sexually active) • I felt calm and sort of joyful • Mum and I went on a 'secret' mission to buy pads •

Women 31-45

At first I was ashamed I'd soiled myself • I hid my undies in my drawer for two months until my mum found them • I showed my mother for confirmation and we jumped around the bathroom • my first period was heralded by incredibly painful cramps that had me doubled over and at the point of vomiting • I saw blood and panicked, it took me a minute to realise what was happening • I thought I was dying. Mum was very reassuring • it was the most exciting day! I was so proud of myself! • I was very sad. I didn't want to be a woman because women are not happy being a woman where I come from • I was MORTIFIED that I had been on public transport and had walked up our big school driveway and through the school with blood all over my dress and no one had told me • we'd had videos at school but I didn't think it would apply to me • I optimistically carried sanitary items in my school bag for three years but was unprepared for the enormity of the pain and sheer volume of blood • I had two older sisters who were very private about their periods but I would sometimes sneak a look in the bathroom bin to suss out what was happening • I had no idea that I would get my period more than once • I had not handled a pad before that day and was sent to school with a thick uncomfortable wad in my undies and was afraid of being 'outed' • the movie Carrie was really popular at the time. It was not a great movie for young girls experiencing puberty • my mom handed me pads and said, 'well, now you can have babies' • I hid my sheets under the bed for a week • I had three periods before mum said anything to me. I didn't know how to bring it up with her • I was a latch key kid scared and alone and I cried for three hours because I didn't know what to do • I had read about it and was very excited but when it actually came I went crying to my mum • I was staying at my dad's house and felt too embarrassed to say anything. Later he told me he had bought pads, but I didn't know that! • my dad was home and I told him. He was really excited and happy for me. He took me inside and sat me down at the table and gave me a small glass of champagne to celebrate • Mum's friend gave me some gemstones in celebration. I felt proud • my brother, who lived in New York and is 15 years older, called and congratulated me! • I named my period Agatha and she became my friend • confused, am I meant to be a woman now? • at last. All I needed now was armpit hair • I received huge congratulations and lots of positive reinforcement • I was watching Sunday Disney and went to the toilet during the ad break and saw the blood in my underwear. I was shocked and frightened • Mum gave me a lovely ceremony with women to celebrate my blood • I used toilet paper for two days then shyly told my mother. She started to cry and handed me some pads. That made me feel worse • Mum had a mixed reaction saying 'wow' and then 'you poor thing'. My dad was excited and proud of me •

Mature women 46 plus

When I first bled Mum gave me a hideous belt, plastic pants and some thick pads and newspaper to wrap them in • I was at my dad's house and I was tackling this ocean of blood with toilet paper as I didn't dare tell him • I didn't tell my mom for a whole year! • beforehand I had a day of writhing around in bed in agony and terror as my mother refused to call the doctor and I couldn't figure out why. Once I got my period she said she'd thought that's what it was • my mother gave me a gift. She was proud of me so I thought it must be a good thing • I had no idea what was happening • panic and shame • I expected some pampering. What I got was some pads and a used sanitary belt • my mother was extremely helpful and gave me great advice • I was stunned to hear about menstruation from a friend in seventh grade. My mother was a nurse and midwife yet still hadn't talked to me about it • my giant of a father went to the store and bought one of each product and gave me the bag • I was terrified. I thought I was dying • I was ashamed. I knew that sex and everything connected with it was BAD • my mother made me go to school, but I bled everywhere, and the embarrassment was awful • when I told Mum there was some blood she gave me a booklet and a brown paper bag with Modess and a belt in it. She never spoke about it again • I cried because I wasn't ready to marry! • I remember 'flooding' in my white jeans. I learnt the hard way about sanitary protection • my mother told me to hide it • I thought I pooped out the wrong hole • coming from a migrant background I thought this was another blight that would add to the prejudice • it scared the heck out of me, I thought I was dying. I went all through the school telling people I was dying • I didn't know what was happening until after I was pregnant with my second child!! I didn't know there was a connection between periods and pregnancy • I thought I must have leukaemia, which had killed my younger brother • I had to have an operation to allow the blood through as I had no vaginal opening. I was told to say it was for my toe when I went back to school • I felt intrigued, somehow magical and powerful • I was happy and got lots of hugs from my mum, and Dad said, 'well done you're a woman'. I was 10! • something between alarm and excitement and insanely private • shattered, ashamed, I did not want or need children, I was not comfortable being female and it made me definitely female • proud that I had finally joined my girlfriends and that I too could talk about 'getting Fred' •

Talking about periods now

Girls 12-15

I'm moody in the week before, I get irrationally annoyed at people • so annoying because you're limited to the activities you can do without it feeling disgusting • it kills, sometimes I have to sit down and curl up into a ball • bothers me a lot because I feel awkward playing sport • annoying sometimes but it means I can have kids when I grow up so it's pretty cool • now I can have babies! • I worry in case someone can see my pad through my pants • I feel as if I can't go to friends places or out in case I leak • ruins my underwear • time consuming, you have to almost plan out your day around it • it just comes and goes and it's fine • it's part of my life and does not bother me. I talk freely to my friends about it • proud •

Girls 16-18

Awful cramps • positive reminder of good health, my body is working the way it is supposed to • after seven years I know exactly what I need in terms of painkillers and size of pads / tampons • it always seems to come at times when I'm really busy and aren't able to take a bit of downtime • frankly, just annoying • my periods make me feel normal and woman-like • I'm on the contraceptive Implanon so I get my period rarely • hate the pain • the pain is the worst part and not knowing when it will come • a relief because I know I'm not pregnant •

Young women 19-30

Cleansing, feminine, healing • I have polycystic ovaries so when I get it I love it! • my periods post-partum have been terrible and PMS dreadful • I used to love getting my period because it made me feel more like a woman, but now it means I'm still not pregnant • I love menstruation and take the time to relax, look inside myself and reflect on the last cycle and thoughts about the next one • I hated it for ages but I always feel better after and it gives me a chance to rest • I try to ignore it and hope it goes away as soon as possible • intense pain on the first day • it feels like someone has taken a hook and attached it to my pelvic region and is running and twisting at the same time • I know it 'could' be a spiritual journey with connection and time for myself, but then I feel guilty when I don't do that • sick, tired and craving chocolate • mellow, reflective, connected to the earth, womanly, deep and ancient, renewed • I've been on the Pill for eight years and just went off it so now I'm quite irregular but feel more myself • tired but energised afterwards • painful, dirty • even if it hurts it's nice to know my body's working and doing its thing • it makes me feel feminine • in bed or trudging for the first few days • glad there's an explanation for my emotional rollercoaster •

Women 31-45

Exhausting but it does give me insight into my body • tedious managing the mess • difficult working with only men • a period means my PMS will end soon • debilitating pain, I don't feel 'right' a lot of the time • the logistics and cost are annoying • it feels dirty • it's my biology, a part of my life • horrendously painful and I get severe migraines • I suffer from PMDD and it's a nightmare • I lose two days a month to pain and mess • it's liberating and feels like a part of womanhood • annoying, but whatever • the best thing is taking codeine to help with cramps and getting all blissed out from that, tbh [too be honest] • I give myself space and more care which has improved my experience • I don't feel supported to take care of myself, and I have to fight to justify, explain and seek permission to retreat every time • its cyclical nature helps guide me, and I love how it works with the moon and my emotions • it interferes with my usual schedule • my children know to give me space and they are gentle with me • I have poor fertility and my period reminds me of this • I enjoy the whole ritual these days •

Mature women 46 plus

Oddly comforting • I don't want to stop and go through menopause • reminds me how fast a month disappears • part of the natural rhythm of life • can't wait for them to stop • my man loves me and will still make love to me which takes the 'tension' I feel away • I have completely changed my appreciation of menses. I enjoy the quiet me-time, cleaning and taking stock mentally, 'being' rather than doing things • I've had it for over 40 years and am ready for it to end • lasts too long and is painful, the emotional stuff is a killer • heavy, crampy and tired • it goes for about ten days – I really need to buy shares in a tampon company • sad as my husband and I will not have any more children • annoying because it is less likely that I will have sex • because of increasing heaviness and pain over the last ten years I have overdosed on strong painkillers • tired and irritable, but once I start to flow, I have a sort of 'cleansing' feeling • PAINFUL, ten days of hell • I feel 100% woman and go with the flow • oh hello, my hormones are still okay • terrible, heavy bleeding and so tired • when will it end? • I rarely have periods now because I have a hormonal IUD so when it turns up it's just annoying • knowing its winding down makes me a little sad • it's very unpredictable • I give my self permission to take it easy and be really kind to myself • I am in peri-menopause and starting to wear my wisdom hat •

Sharing about the influence of family

Young women 19-30

When I first got my period my Dad said something like 'oh great, another in the house' • the way my mother talked made it sound like the plague! • when I got my first period we had a party, although I didn't understand then why it was special or important, I do now • my dad gave me a very cute congratulations on the first day of my first period saying it was like getting your first grey hair – not something you wanted but a great sign you were maturing • mum was very open about menstruation and sexual education • my mum didn't know what to do with me • it was always easy to talk about • I grew up with an ob/gyn so it's just a fact of life • I live in a sexist, male-run family. It makes it difficult • in my culture getting your period meant you became a 'señorita', which meant you weren't a child anymore. I felt resistant as I didn't want to stop being a kid • I live with my dad now, he buys me tampons, makes me hot water bottles and listens to me complain • my family did not and do not discuss it. No one I know has pain and heavy bleeding like me • my mom congratulated me and told me she loved me and that I'm a woman now • menstruation is looked upon as embarrassing and shameful by some of the men in my family and this is the source of the shame and embarrassment I feel for my feminine body and being • I didn't even disclose that I had my period for six months. I think the poor communication in my family has significantly contributed to my inability to accept menstruation as a normal part of life • my mom was sexually abused as an adolescent and then became a psychologist, so she really wanted my sister and I to be knowledgeable about our bodies. I was a little shy about all the information as a child but now, as a mother of three, I love being connected and in tune with my body and cycles • my mother never said anything about periods and she does not till this day • I grew up with my grandfather and he was not understanding at all and often made me feel embarrassed • my grandmother was a postpartum nurse for 35 years so she helped me understand what it was and what I could do to feel better • I was raised Jewish and I have three aunts. There was a lot of feminism and Goddess empowerment in my childhood. I was given so many books about what to expect from puberty. We went to dinner to celebrate my first menstruation • in my family it is something to be managed with pain medication, keeping clean and making sure you don't smell • when I first got my period I was really bad at controlling leaks and remembering to change my pads. My mother would always get really mad when I stained my underwear, so I sometimes hid them under my bed • my family has never spoken about menstruation – I had to figure it out for myself •

Women 31-45

In my family it was a curse, so when I first got my period even though I was excited I didn't share it • in my Indian culture getting your period is a step into womanhood, so everyone knows and everyone celebrates • Mum gave me pads to hide in my drawer away from my father and brother • it was treated as a day to dread • my father's lewd comments about women impacted greatly on my feelings about myself and how I felt as a woman, including about menstruation • the men in my family were well educated about menstruation and were sensitive to women's issues • my mother gave me books and tried to talk about it but she was still full of shame • growing up in a traditional Jewish household, it was more about keeping clean and not being allowed to kiss the Torah • my mother made me feel ashamed for wanting to use tampons • everything about sex was negative in my family so I thought my body was dirty and shameful • I felt that if my mom couldn't talk about it there must be something very wrong • my mother had a highly negative perspective about being a woman. She hated menstruation and said women are damned to bleed 'like pigs' • Mom made a point of celebrating my menarche by buying me a card and an earring and jewellery box set that I still have. This had a huge impact and I've always been comfortable talking about it • I picked up from a very young age that the male gender was superior, the female weak • Sri Lankan families celebrate periods starting with a party, with ALL YOUR FAMILY THERE • Mum always uses diminutive forms or silly synonyms for intimate parts of life. This has made it feel like I should not take anything seriously that has to do with being a woman • I grew up with two brothers who teased me all the time about my body • Mom was incredibly open and positive about my period and all my body changes. Because of her wonderful attitude I had no fear of menstruation. I have incredibly painful cramps and severe bloating but still feel a reverence towards my cycle • I was not allowed to feel unwell around my period and it had to be really painful for me to get any empathy • a very open mum. I would watch her insert tampons as she chatted away • culturally there are a lot of taboos around periods in India. I have only just begun to feel more positive after having my son. I look at him and think if not for the 'unclean burden' I would not have been able to have him • Mum was excited when I first had it. Dad even more so • my older brother asked me all about it when he started dating girls and we covered the whole topic including tampons • conflicting messages: bleeding is what it means to be a woman, but DO NOT UNDER ANY CIRCUMSTANCES TALK ABOUT IT • I learned a lot of shame about the female body from my mother. Unravelling this shame has been a major project •

Mature women 46 plus

I was taught that menstruation, menopause and childbearing would make me vulnerable and vulnerability equals weakness • my parents celebrated when I got my first period. My mother told me her father pampered her when she had hers • it was not discussed despite my father being a GP • I grew up with my mother and five sisters so our experiences were NORMAL and spoken about openly • my family didn't talk about it, which made me feel not okay being a girl • I have a very open relationship with my dad and he was the first person I told the morning I found I had my first period • I was told repeatedly it was 'the curse' and felt cursed for having it • there were comments like 'we'll have to watch her now. She can get pregnant' as if I was some kind of whore • my religious upbringing devalued all things feminine • I am deeply grateful that I received knowledge of my feminine body at home with my mother, grandmothers and great-grandmothers • everything to do with sex, reproduction and bodily functions was 100% taboo • my family were hard workers and saw slowing down as shirking so I had to soldier on, even when I had bad pain, heavy bleeding and would occasionally faint. It was just part of the burden of being a woman • Mum seemed to relate menstruation to girls being vulnerable to sexual assault • even though my mother had seven children she could never talk about anything to do with the body • despite being told 'you can talk to us about anything' when I had my first period I was fobbed off with no explanation and told to go to my room until I stopped crying • I was shamed and ridiculed by my father. I suffered from very severe PMS most of my life • I have never forgotten the time my mother insisted I lie to my friend about why I couldn't go swimming. I couldn't understand what was wrong with speaking the truth • my mother's information and pad pack ready in my bag made it all smooth when I got my period – I felt very comfortable talking to her • my dad was religious and told us that labour and menstruation were God's punishment for Eve's sin in the garden of Eden. My mom countered this by telling us it was simply nature and how we evolved as humans. This left some cognitive dissonance, but the influence of my mom was much stronger • I grew up with eight brothers and seven sisters. Half the population in the house was female and yet there was not one pad or tampon in sight • my family is good about menopause. It was a time for me to really journey into myself and find my own inner peace •

Thoughts on intimate partners, menstruation and menopause

I've had boyfriends who were not understanding and only focused on the negative aspects, like moodiness, and this whole 'gosh you women are so emotional' schtick. But I've also had a boyfriend who was super straightforward • I resent the fact that so many men are 'repulsed' or 'disgusted'. There were times I was made to feel I should be apologetic because I had my period • my partner grew up to believe that women were unclean when they had their period. Fortunately, he no longer believes this • I really appreciate my partner's compassion and understanding at different stages of my cycle, like when I'm exhausted and irritable • once I was going home with a guy and was like, 'I can't sleep with you, I'm on my period' and he was just so chill about it • I don't feel as though I can have sexual intercourse when I have my period. I think my partner would think it's unclean • my husband is very supportive and knowledgeable about periods and our two daughters talk freely too • I love the feeling of acceptance of my womanhood that making love during my period brings • my husband and son are very supportive – they are the only ones in my long life who have been • my boyfriend is lovely and supportive about me being in pain and wants to comfort me but I can tell he finds periods gross in general, even though he tries to hide it • my husband does not fully understand what having my period means in terms of the impact on my body. His family is English and very uncommunicative about all personal matters, so menstruation was never mentioned while he was growing up • my now ex-husband often made reference to my mood swings as being 'psychopathic'. In hindsight I think this is a cruel label for me and other women struggling with their natural body clock • I am so drained by conversations with my partner where my very real feelings are dismissed as being 'hormonal', that is, less valid. I believe it's almost at the biological and spiritual heart of misogyny • menopause crept up slowly, so it wasn't too bad. The worst was how my now ex-husband had absolutely no appreciation of women's issues and no interest in trying to understand • when I was experiencing menopause I was married to a man who was very selfish, who gave me no support. I was stressed and depressed •

Reflecting on the experience of having periods at work

My functioning at work is significantly affected by periods. This is so taboo! My managers have mostly been women and there is no way they would acknowledge periods or women's functioning as cyclical • I feel a pressure to carry on as normal when I suffer quite badly and am often unable to do this • I have great understanding from my boss, though he is uncomfortable with the topic so I 'don't feel well' once a month • I'm angry that some women don't have pain and suffering during periods and think those who do are faking it to get out of work! • on some occasions I am legitimately very unwell where I require a day off work but feel unable to be honest about this because of the stigma attached to being 'weak' or 'a princess' for not being able to cope with it. This forces me lie to my employer • I love being a woman and know my rhythms well. But living and working in a world that does not respect this makes it so difficult for me • even in all-female, feminist workplaces it still feels very hidden •

Difficulties managing periods at work

When I was working I had to frequently go to the toilet every one-and-a-half to two hours as the flow was so heavy • I felt my workplace was judgmental and unsympathetic to the levels of tiredness and mood changes I experienced – it added to my performance scrutiny stress • going to the toilet every two hours to change a pad or tampon was obvious to everyone and was seen as time-wasting • I had a spell of flooding during peri-menopause which made me feel self-conscious at work • my male manager was NOT understanding and suggested I take a MLOA (Medical Leave of Absence) every month because I had heavy bleeding and needed to work from home • I still feel I have to 'tough it out' if I have a heavy bleed • I find it very hard to concentrate during menstruation because I get headaches and visual-disturbance migraines. I have an academic job, which requires a lot of focus, and I also find meetings difficult • I have a demanding job as an OR RN and do try to stay home if I know I cannot make it through thirteen focused hours on my feet. Luckily, I work three days per week and ask my body to time it well so I can give it what it needs. Often works! • I'd like to feel free to use a heat pad at work and not have to hide a tampon to go to the bathroom. And, to never again hear a man accuse my bad mood on my period • I'm angry that some women don't have pain and suffering during periods and think those who do are faking it to get out of work! • going to the toilet every two hours to change a pad or tampon was obvious to everyone and seen as time wasting • on some occasions I'm very unwell and need a day off work, but feel unable to be honest about it because of the stigma attached to being 'weak' or 'a princess' for not being able to cope. This forces me lie to my employer • I love being a woman and know my rhythms well. But living and working in a world that does not respect this makes it so difficult for me • even in all-female, feminist workplaces it still feels very hidden • my GP was helpful when I told her that I couldn't tolerate having to work with multiple changes of pads and tampons per shift •

Being self-employed and managing periods

I am lucky to be self-employed, so I make sure I take the time to slow down and reflect during my bleed time • being self-employed, I take the time I need for myself. I am eager to tell other women how easy it can be and how to make it that way • there were days at work when I nearly passed out, my colleagues just laughed • I was very fortunate to be on sabbatical while going through menopause – I think the transitioning actually enhanced the work I was doing at the time; fortunately I was able to set my own schedule, e.g. it helped to be able to sleep in if I'd been awake for a while early in the morning and I was able to cry as much or as often as it came up •

Negative attitudes to menstruation and menopause in the workplace

There is a tendency to shame women who don't disguise the fact that they are experiencing menstruation or menopause. There is also the attitude that 'hormonal' women don't function well in the work place, which makes women feel they have to hide what is happening. I once sat in a city business meeting where one of the other women apologised for the fact that I had had a hot flush then handed the decision we were making over to the only man present 'as we were all middle aged and hormonal' as she thought he would make the decision better • it's often used in a way to make women out to be 'too emotional' and 'illogical' when there is a real problem they are trying to communicate • unhelpful comment from a male work colleague: 'PMS does not actually exist' • the mood swings made it impossible in the workplace to retain any dignity • woman are expected to function the same at work during this time, ridiculous! Society has little information on menopause • I have had days at work when I've felt exhausted, due to sleepless nights • I have greatly disliked having to work and be busy at this time and now I plan around it as much as possible • I didn't have any discernible medical reason for the extreme pain and nausea I experience – trying to get employers to understand that this is real, severe and not made up is exasperating • I feel that these days women are expected to behave like men and not admit to feeling differently at different times in their cycle. It is feminism gone askew! • I was on the birth control Pill for two years when I was a virgin. How dare my employer slut shame me for using medication to help my menstrual condition • too many men will, if you disagree with them, say, 'What, are you on the rag or somethin'?!' What a great way for men to belittle women – especially in the workplace! •

Managing symptoms of peri-menopause and menopause at work

I did not have a bad time but my sleep was very disrupted and so I was often dragged out at work during the day. Having the opportunity to work part-time or set my own hours and work from home would have helped a lot • I am peri-menopausal and struggling with how hot my body is! I wish the company I work for were more accommodating of menopausal women. I am worried that I won't cope • looking forward to being done with the mental roller coaster of peri-menopause. My employers are from the 'suck it up and get over it' school • peri-menopause was awful – heavy bleeding made teaching difficult. I was unable to make a quick exit to the bathroom when necessary • I am dreading getting red and hot in business meetings in my male-dominated technical field • I felt I couldn't tell anyone that I had a hysterectomy and made something up about why I couldn't be at work •

On the loss of privacy and dignity when menstruating at work

Several months ago, on the first day of my period I was in a meeting at work and the cramps built to the point I nearly passed out. I left the meeting because I couldn't function, and a female co-worker came to help and eventually I found myself back at my cube, which I share with a guy. At that point I had to talk openly about what was going on and that I might need his help to go to the ER because I was so lightheaded. I suddenly felt very exposed and vulnerable, having shared a level of personal information that I try to keep out of the workplace. However, he's a good friend and his focus was only on getting me help if I needed it and that helped me feel less ashamed • I don't like all of the jokes and negativity around menstruation, especially when it comes from men • please may I never again hear a man accuse my bad mood on my period • I really dislike the way men feel 'grossed out' when they hear or see anything about periods – it's not a thing to be ashamed of •

Speaking about menstruation, menopause and health care

On difficulties in getting appropriate health care

My mother let me stay home from school because of the agonizing pain I had each period. Sometimes I would need three days off though she never thought to take me to a doctor about it • my periods are erratic and last for over a month. I have tried nearly every option and of those I haven't it's because of their side effects or contraindications • I could not manage it without the Pill. I get diarrhoea, low blood pressure, extreme dizziness and acne when I'm not on the Pill. I've also attended Emergency Departments for excessive bleeding • my mother really should have sought medical help for me but would have been too embarrassed to take me to our GP who was male and a neighbour. My symptoms were so extreme that it was impossible to hide them from my father who decided that I willed it on myself. He eventually came to realise that this was not the case •

On appreciating periods despite having menstrual problems

Having PCOS and fertility problems has made me appreciate menstruation much more and it would be nice if women felt empowered by the amazing miracle that their body performs each month, rather than feeling ashamed or dirty or embarrassed • in my early twenties I discovered I had PCOS. After seeing a naturopath and a chiropractor I was able to heal. I have a regular cycle now but I still feel that I am consistently working hard at my health and keeping PCOS at bay, at being conscious of my emotions, hormones, and my thoughts and how they affect my body. I am so thankful for my period and my body now and have so much more respect and love for them • when my periods stopped my doctor said congratulations! I asked her if it was a problem and her response was do you know how many women wish they could stop theirs? That's when I stopped taking the Pill and took charge of my own hormonal health. I needed to know how my body was being affected by my diet, my surroundings, environmental and emotional, and I found that my menstrual cycle was a great gauge •

APPENDIX TWO

On cyclic mental health impacts

I was diagnosed at 30 with PMDD. This is a far worse problem than bleeding. When your mind is messed up, your entire life is turned upside down. I took medication for 20 years (Prozac) and it helped IMMENSELY • learning to respect and work with my cycle rather than pushing myself through it has been one of the tools that has helped me to heal from depression • I really loath and despise the prevalent discourse around PMS and the suggestion that it is a mental pathology (DSM-V). It seems as though PMS is another flaw that keeps women somehow at a lower level than rational, noncyclical men in the very patriarchal medical and mental-health profession discourse • there isn't enough information, research or support for people who suffer PMDD, so people who have it mostly suffer in silence and shame. It's really awful • I want to feel the power of my stronger feelings during menstruation without being overcome by them • I am still trying to figure out how to balance my premenstrual experience which can feel pretty extreme, especially emotionally • when I get PMS, I see it like a veil of social correctness has dropped and I can listen to what is lurking underneath. So, if I'm angry I can tap into what is making me angry and work on that, or sad, or whatever • the more open we are with others and particularly our friends and children, the better. Not just the physical 'facts' but emotional honesty about all that menstruation brings • I have had problems with depression that I have only recently begun to correlate to my hormones – early when my period first began, and for the past 20 years – I had my first post-partum depression after the birth of my last child then continued on into peri-menopause. I am sure there are many more like me but it is not something widely acknowledged or accepted • I wish I wouldn't bleed so much: clothes, bed, carpet – all stained. I take a towel with me to the movie theatre to sit on, so I don't have 'an accident'. I've done this to myself with negative thinking habits, mostly wanting to be dead to escape. If I can get a handle on my life, I can turn things around, I can stop the alarming amount of blood loss •

On the positive and negative impacts of visiting health practitioners

I am so discouraged by medical clinicians that say PMS does not exist. They should try living in my body/brain the week before my period for the last thirty years! • I wish more doctors understood the importance of regular menstrual cycles and were more sensitive to women who do not menstruate regularly • I don't like the way doctors dismiss what you're experiencing, even women • I wish my endometriosis had been diagnosed in my teen years rather than having suffered through such cramps and heavy periods for so long. I thought the excruciating monthly pain was normal. It was my normal, but I didn't know what normal was • male doctors should be more compassionate and not focus on getting rid of women's ovaries when they're going into menopause just to make money • my male GYNE was very quick to recommend a hysterectomy, saying 'You don't need it'. I said, 'I will be the judge of that' • I bled heavily and randomly from my first period to my last. For two years during my late twenties I bled every day and was frequently dismissed by doctors, especially males. I was told to have more babies to regulate my period! I was eventually diagnosed with endometriosis and underwent a hysterectomy at 33, thank goodness! • I wish doctors were more informed. One said it was all in my head • my daughter had very heavy periods and was put on two sorts of Pill. One made her weepy and unhappy, and with the other she became light sensitive and had double vision – they thought it might be a blood clot. I was furious that the medical system pops young women on the Pill without first considering a holistic approach. She cured herself with yoga and gym and by changing her diet and getting off the computer more often • I wish our gynes were more informed and not drug dealers! And that they wouldn't reprimand us for NOT taking their drugs • since the birth of my first child when I was 23, I have had very heavy periods with a lot of clotting and pain and every doctor I have discussed this with says 1. it's normal and 2. if it bothers me that much I should get a hysterectomy. Neither option is an acceptable medical opinion IMO! • I had to join an online group in order to talk to someone who understood what I was going through. My doctor was somewhat dismissive and did not have time to really talk to me about menopause • I was on HRT for years. It kept my energy down and it was like I had chronic fatigue and depression. When I stopped I recovered my energy and myself. My local doctor discouraged me and said that I was irresponsible • I had very heavy bleeding during peri-menopause and my M.D. at the time suggested a hysterectomy, but I found a naturopath covered by my insurance and she assured me that all was normal. I had few other symptoms and feel great in menopause • doctors thought I had a kidney infection, my husband suggested it may be a mental condition. It wasn't until I saw a new Chinese woman doctor, who didn't have the preconceived ideas that prevail with Western male doctors, that menopause was finally diagnosed and found to be well advanced • helps to have a terrific female Dr who discusses all of the likely effects/experiences freely and openly. Makes me confident that menopausal changes can be dealt with as and when they arise • I did not really understand the extent to which menopause would affect my sex life. When I spoke to a male doctor about a lack of sex drive he said 'oh well you have had all your children now so it shouldn't be an issue'! • years of painful periods in spite of various treatments, followed by a dreadful time in my forties with very heavy bleeding due to fibroids which became constant and in spite of being very reluctant I had a radical hysterectomy aged 49. Within weeks I felt a new woman and although my menopause symptoms have been fairly uncomfortable I wouldn't have my periods back for anything • it helps to have a terrific female Dr who discusses all of the likely effects and experiences freely and openly. Makes me confident that menopausal changes can be dealt with as and when they arise •

On finding relief from symptoms

Even though I have fibroids and heavy bleeding now there have been many times where I have loved having my period and the heightened creativity, insight and feelings of oneness that it bestows • wish I had a better idea about how nutrition impacted the experience when I was younger. Have no doubt that systemic candida and other issues made my cycles a living hell • exercise, caffeine-free, healthy diet made an incredible difference to my periods and menopause • my naturopath advised me to take sage steeped in lemon juice daily for two weeks to help the hot flushes. It worked a treat! •

Living with a disability and how this impacts periods

Very hard when I can't walk normally • with an anxiety disorder my periods are sometimes off-schedule because of intense stress • I have Lyme disease with multiple co-infections. My periods cause inflammation levels to rise which makes most of my symptoms worse for the whole period • I have vision impairment, so I don't always know when I have my period, whether I am dripping blood around bathrooms and whether I have been able to clean clothes and sheets enough so the blood's not visible • it does not except for the gendered assumptions in these questions • the body awareness issues that come with Autism Spectrum Disorder have been challenging. I don't necessarily pick up the subtle 'period coming!' signs my body gives out as well as neurotypical women would. Also, people with ASD can be less than brilliant at hygiene the best of times, which feeds into my paranoia about cleanliness • I have depression, anxiety, trouble sleeping and endometriosis, which causes lots of pain and makes it harder to sleep. The cyclic hormone changes make managing my mental health difficult and my mental health also affects my ability to maintain proper hygiene. I also have long periods • I can't use tampons, so I sometimes get infections from my vagina/vulva not being able to breath • mine is a mental illness (depression) but I don't feel it impacts my experience of periods. I have come to terms with my body and all of its emissions! • hormonal mood swings make my depression worse and sometimes scares me • periods definitely make my depression worse • I don't think it does • no effect • I am always worried about period stains in my white cricket pants • it does not • I have had much more difficulty understanding what was happening, learning how to manage it and getting support to learn those things than other women • my disability has nothing to do with my experience of menstruation • my disability wasn't apparent until I was 40 • not at all – my disability (mild acquired brain injury) was acquired approximately six months before menopause • my physical disability came later • I have had rheumatoid arthritis, diagnosed at seventeen. Fortunately, it only started to limit me five years ago. C'est la vie. I do feel the corticosteroids affected my emotional state in the long term, but I cannot link those swings exclusively to PMS •

Speaking about the prospect and experience of menopause

On the prospect of menopause

Looking forward to it! • sad no more prospect of babies! Happy to not have the rollercoaster ride of hormones during the menstrual cycle and peri-menopause! • trepidation, I'm ready to stop bleeding but not ready for the accompanying hormonal changes and the transformation into an old person! • unsure, hope it's not too topsy turvy • not looking forward to it! Feel like I have just got my head together and am a bit daunted knowing that it is inevitable • excited! • am just starting to have hot flushes and night sweats which are far more of an issue than my period ever was • excited but also nervous – I feel so young still – looking forward to what develops in my harvest time • a little anxious because menstruation has been sacred for me • I have lost one third of my life to menstrual pain and suffering for the past 37 years and I can't wait for this to be over • am a bit worried about ailments and am already experiencing mood swings reminiscent of my menarche, 'holy rage' I call it • I want to find role models who have been able to happily maintain their marriage/relationship through menopause • HAPPY!!! • scared • bring it on! Except for the growing old part • excited!!!!!! • sad to leave this stage of fertility, eager to be done with heavy painful periods • much as I dislike periods I like that afterwards I feel light and energetic. I am fearful of the new set of issues that will come with it • I will mourn the loss of regular periods. I'm hopeful that my sex drive will stick around and I'm looking forward to not riding the hormonal roller coaster as much • positive but hate the embarrassing hot flushes and mood swings! • looking forward to no more drainage from my body and not panicking about access to sanitary products and toilets • not looking forward to it as I am recently divorced, and I think it reduces women's attractiveness to men! Though it will be a relief not to have to worry about pregnancy and miscarriages • ambivalent – my cycle is so much a part of me • talking with other women about it is really helpful • a little sad, I would have liked to have another baby but too late • scared about the loss of fertility and my identity that's wrapped up in my reproductive potential • now that I am so enjoying my menstruation I am a little tentative about giving it up at menopause! • yes, please! And, hurry up! Anything to stop the constant bleeding • YAAAAAAAAY! • looking forward to it although, after many years of harrowing menstruation, I now enjoy having a period • not looking forward to it because I enjoy knowing my body is still young enough to be able to menstruate • I know it's next and normal but I'm a bit sad • the sooner the better • I would rather menstruate • fucking HATE it. It makes me feel really old. I'm VERY depressed about it • looking forward to being done bleeding at 50, I feel sexier and more alive than ever • I'd like to delay it as long as possible • like it's the final kick in teeth to being a girl • another natural progression of life •

APPENDIX TWO

On anxiety and concern

I feel like it will immediately age me ten years • even though I have no desire to have more children, the reality of the finality of that choice did make me feel a little sad • sad to live the later years without the hormones that make me a woman: dry skin, dry hair, grey cloud/depression days, allergies • hope that my hormonal fluctuations will even out and I will regain a sense of consistent energy • I did not have babies yet and my heart still wants them • mixed feelings. I won't miss periods but have to accept I'm not 'young' any more • worried that menopause will speed the aging process, i.e. sagging skin and hair loss • worried about the effect on mood and memory • sad. It seems to be the end of an era. I want to maintain my youth and vitality. I am concerned about the negative impact on my body • worried that it might be overwhelming or that I might lose my sex drive or get really cranky • feels like the end of all those chances to have a baby – more grief! • nervous, excited, hope I don't shrivel up and become unattractive and lose my sex appeal and desire • dread it – I will be old! • I was a little sad when I realised it's HIGHLY unlikely my lover and I will conceive. Otherwise I'm not upset except for the weight gain around my middle and fatigue • I'm struggling with how hot my body is!! I wish the company I work for was more accommodating for menopausal women. I am worried that I won't cope with menopause! • I was concerned about various aspects of my hormones and lack of sex drive so went on hormone replacement therapy. But it hurt my breasts and it frightened me, so I stopped. I began to do more yoga, massage and meditation to balance myself. This has worked for me • looking forward to being done with the mental roller coaster of peri-menopause. My husband is from the 'suck it up and get over it' school, as are employers. Talk about a mid-life crisis :) •

On looking forward to menopause

I'm hoping it brings some relief from the effects of endometriosis • looking forward to it as a sign of my next phase in life • I CAN'T WAIT!!!! I am going to have the biggest party • now that I have a teenager and too many subsequent miscarriages I am past being a new mother. I will feel like my body has caught up to my state of mind • looking forward to a new chapter in my life • delighted and excited ready to be done with the bleeding and to move into crone • this period of life exciting and am re-evaluating of my life and what I want. It almost feels like a second adolescence! • mixed, but I intend to take proactive measures with my health and wellness • can't wait but wish bioidenticals [hormone therapy] were more readily available and less expensive • it's a natural thing that will come and I embrace it • hope to be able to go through this life phase with the help of natural remedies and no hormones. I am also excited and hope to become a wiser, more grounded and loving person when all this has passed • feeling fine and am starting to read and study as much as I can. Knowing that it is a very individual thing I prepare by maintaining a level of fitness and nutrition • honoured to enter the circle of the wise women and step into a new chapter of my life • being a grandmother now, I look forward to menopause • I like that this phase can be very empowering • wildly freeing, very sacred doorway to intuition explosion!! Wise years, my hair is a beautiful grey already • defiant, I look fifteen years plus younger now so I'm going with that theme. A bit of freedom will be great without having to deal with the monthly issues • I welcome peri-menopause and view impending menopause as an empowering new stage in my life • feeling good: menopause is a transition that is empowering, it brings a quiet fire to put yourself first • I am also a little excited about crone-hood •

On finding useful information

I would like to have more info on how to treat menopause naturally and holistically • thrilled! Reading has helped me to understand what a great time it can be, the beginning of the second half of my life • having just done a menopause workshop I feel much excitement at the prospect of menopause and the phase of life after. It also educated me on the self-care I need to be doing now • I wish women talked about menopause and what to expect more. I've had trouble finding information on how to negotiate it •

On real life experiences of menopause

It is unremittingly 'the change' but I chose to experience it as a Rite of Passage, as a path to deep healing, self-love and compassion • at 48 I was prescribed implants to shrink fibroids prior to a hysterectomy. It was a very sudden transition • I enjoy having a more even keel, less emotional ups and downs and not having to worry about pregnancy or painful periods • I feel like my femininity has been taken away. The hot flushes and dehydration just about do me in. I hate having to be medicated just to get through the day • I don't miss bleeding or cramps but don't like the total loss of libido and weight gain • I have found connections, education and women's circles to help me navigate this time, with love, respect and curiosity • I feel liberated! I feel much healthier and alive, don't suffer from premenstrual headaches and mood swings, and am motivated to complete projects • hot flashes have been an annoying presence for ten years. I wonder if something is so wrong with my thermostat now and it will never correct itself • night sweats and lack of sleep are really hard, especially working at the same time • unbearable hot flushes, very poor sleep, low libido but no more periods. Yay! • very little information on the positive only the negative • other than it means I'm older this has been the best time of my life because my periods were so awful • menopause ROCKS! It is awesome brain chemistry! • doing the VERY happy dance! • being able to stay on one emotional level for weeks and months I became clear and was able to get myself out of a terrible situation • am finally beginning to feel like my old self but went through about five years of emotional and physical hell • do miss the hormones as I see my skin turning to crepe and my libido disappearing. I do like the stability and clarity though, and the delight of gaining wisdom and becoming a better person • most challenging for me was the realization of no more babies :) • hormonal changes caused my anxiety and insomnia to skyrocket • I want all my eggs and all those painful periods back • free at last!!!!!!!!!!!!!!!!!! • I like not having to worry about getting pregnant • the positive is the acceptance of self that comes once you understand what this life stage means but the symptoms have been horrendous • I miss the effects of oestrogen like nice skin • I have a group of girlfriends who are very supportive and chat about menopause freely and with great cheer • I suffered badly. Getting the right treatment took years • I couldn't understand why it wasn't talked about more, and why I hadn't really known about this impact on so many women • uncomfortable, fat and HOT • there were days at work when I nearly passed out and colleagues just laughed • connecting to a new space, new identity and new energy however I am disappointed at the culture in Australia around 'older' women, which does not reflect my personal sense of wisdom • extreme hot flushes accompanied by distressing panic attacks. I thought I was going insane until I spoke to a girlfriend who experienced the same thing • had a spell of flooding during peri-menopause which made me feel very self-conscious at work • I likened perimenopause to the last trimester of pregnancy, only instead of a baby being born, I WAS BORN, me the grown-up WOMAN •

What Women Told Us Would Help

Girls talk about what would make things better at school

Not having to be careful about it being obvious to people who don't know • not having to worry about whether or not there's a bin • not having to say I'm sick when I can't go swimming no danger of leakage • being allowed to go outside for a bit or being able to go to the toilet whenever • having a day off when I have cramps would be nice but I don't actually like missing school • silent wrappers so other girls won't know and tell the boys • not getting teased by the boys • not being afraid that someone will see me getting a tampon from my bag • I wish that people wouldn't think it such a private thing, so then I could explain why I was sharp with them or suddenly wince in pain • soundless pad wrappers • for people not to laugh about periods • more pockets in my clothing to put pads in • more talks to help inform me and other people on how to help with periods • don't make fun of me!! • with almost chronic period pains I always need days off which means I lie about being sick or something. I wish I didn't have to • if periods weren't seen as a disgusting thing it would be much easier to manage as you wouldn't need to plan everything in advance and no need for stupid cover up excuses • acceptance and tolerance from males, even females • no more PMS jokes! • if guys and girls were more open about it, it would be way less awkward • Women talk about the consequences of their lack of education Emotional support in the early years would have had a profound effect on my self-image! • in my 30s I bought myself books that I wish I had when I was ten to thirteen that talk about our bodies. I promised myself I would retrain my thirteen-year-old self with proper information • its annoying how sometimes while menstruating I feel sad and angry and my mood changes drastically and I don't know how to control it. It makes me mad and I feel I lack education on the subject • I'd love to see girls be taught about how to deal with the symptoms of period pain and PMS – no one warned me that I would feel like I was getting stabbed in the uterus or that I would literally cry over spilt milk • I'd like to see it talked about more in spaces like schools, shopping centres and women's spaces – there are so many questions around it and so little public and open discussion • start educating boys about menstruation. They're taught at a young age by macho apes to crack jokes about periods, and to demean and disregard women because of this natural process. Too many men will, if you disagree with them, say, 'What, are you on the rag or somethin'?!' • we need to educate our daughters to not be ashamed of talking about their period. To also educate our sons that it's natural and a beautiful part of being a woman •

When a deliberately positive menstrual culture is created at home

My husband is totally cool with buying tampons. I only heard him complain once that all the bathrooms in the house are menstruation infested. I guess that's what happens with all girls and a full moon ;-) • very open about my period with my girls and daughters-in-law and we discuss them in front of my boys and sons-in-law. They're all getting used to it :) • my husband is very supportive and knowledgeable about periods and our two daughters talk freely too • I married an Indian whose female relatives were very talkative and supportive and told me not to feel 'shamed'!! • when my daughter got her first period I was at work and her older brother got her a hot water bottle and made her lie down as she had pain, he then rang me to say she was okay • Mom never talked about it and I had a horrible experience at menarche and won't repeat that with my ten year old daughter;) • I have a family history of gynaecological problems and shame; mum had endometriosis so was in pain all the time, I have PCOS so my period is unpredictable. I've tried very hard to celebrate it with my daughter – in particular the power to create life, which is pretty cool • Mum was very embarrassed talking about it with me though we talk freely about menstruation now. I am very open with my daughter and gave her a menarche ceremony when she first bled • I am the mother of three teenage daughters and we openly discuss everything. My husband sometimes finds this confronting however he gets the importance of sharing information and over time has become more accepting and knowledgeable about female anatomy • I have two boys that I have talked to about how natural and normal it is for a woman to bleed each month – nothing to fear or be ashamed or embarrassed about • my family background has made me determined to be open and honest with both my daughter and son • I was taught periods were something women just have to deal. I am trying to change this with my daughters. I would like them to be proud and welcoming of their moontime • if I have a daughter, I will be very open with her, talking about menstruation and puberty from an early age •

Changes women would like to see in workplace menstrual culture

It was considered a normal part of women's lives and normal that we take one or two days off to take care of ourselves • we lived in a fair society where women would be able to take time off to bleed. It's emotionally draining and physically painful and should be accommodated • rest was mandatory. The period flows better and so much emotional turmoil in the world could be avoided if a woman can nurture her body at this time. Modern life does not always make space for this • I'd had the opportunity to work part-time, or set my own hours and work from home some days, as my sleep was very disturbed and I was dragged out during the day during peri-menopause • it were okay to say you have bad menstrual cramps to an employer without them feeling uncomfortable • I felt free to use a heat pad at work and not have to hide a tampon to go to the bathroom. And, to never again hear a man accuse my bad mood on my period • the company I work for were more accommodating of menopausal women. I am peri-menopausal and struggling with how hot my body is! • I could speak about it without whispering. My employer is really good, but I would like other employees to be more vocal. No more silence! I'm tired of hiding my pads • we had menstrual leave • women and girls had more time off and consideration from employers for what we go through •

Menstruation for self-employed women

I am lucky to be self-employed, so I make sure I take the time to slow down and reflect during my bleed time • if I have to rest, I can work my day around it • I take the time I need for myself. I'm eager to tell other women how easy it can be and how to make it that way. I always correct people who make fun of menopause's effects on women and inform those who are ignorant of what a great time it can be if you learn to embrace it rather than fight it • I greatly dislike having to work and be busy at this time, so I plan around it as much as possible •

About creativity, productivity and the menstrual cycle

I've always wished it was something more celebrated and recognised as the powerful event it is, rather than an irritating inconvenience that slows down the work expected of me • the more that I dive into menstrual awareness for my self the more that I am moved to honour the masculine and help men find their true power also. Women – and men too! – need to be taught from the start about the importance of the female's natural cycle, to celebrate and honour this, and to adapt life to work around the female cycle, rather than it being viewed as an inconvenience to have to deal with • I noticed that menstruation affects me more if I don't use my creative energy well around ovulation time •

Women share their experiences and ideas about health care

On visiting doctors with menstrual problems

I am so discouraged by medical clinicians that say PMS does not exist. They should try living in my body / brain the week before my period for the last thirty years! • it's difficult to find a GP who actively discusses the range of symptoms and a range of treatments. Some treatments are so simple and natural, but the information is hard and costly to access • I have a terrific female Dr who discusses all of the likely effects/experiences freely and openly. Makes me confident that menopausal changes can be dealt with as and when they arise • I took charge of my own life and rested when I needed to. But MD's seem to believe this is a disease process and not a natural one • accurate and complete information from my doctors would have been helpful • more reliable support from my gynaecologist and physician about natural treatments would have been appreciated • my GP was sadly behind the times so I did my own research • my experience has been that Western doctors don't appreciate the importance of hormonal balance, how to diagnose and find the cause of imbalance and how to restore and maintain balance naturally without harmful side effects • I bled heavily and randomly from my first period to my last. For two years during my late twenties I bled every day and was frequently dismissed by Drs, especially males. I was told to have more babies to regulate my period! I was eventually diagnosed with endometriosis and underwent a hysterectomy at 33 • my GP was helpful when I told her that I couldn't tolerate having to work with multiple changes of pads and tampons per shift •

On finding what helped

I found that if I eat healthily PMS symptoms are greatly diminished • I wish more therapies like Maya abdominal massage and herbs were offered to women. These approaches can really help women have a better experience of menstruation and menopause • diet, cleansing and meditation plus increased self-awareness and exploration has had a positive influence on my experience of menstruation and now the early stages of menopause • wish I had a better idea about how nutrition impacted the experience when I was younger. Have no doubt that systemic candidas and other issues made my cycles a living hell • exercise and a caffeine free, healthy diet made an incredible difference to my periods and menopause • my naturopath advised me to take sage steeped in lemon juice daily for two weeks to help the hot flushes. It worked a treat! • natural (Chinese) medicine saw me through menopause without any side effects • in my early twenties I discovered I had PCOS. After seeing a naturopath and a chiropractor I was able to heal and have a regular cycle now. Though I'm still working hard at my health and keeping PCOS at bay, at being conscious of my emotions, hormones, and my thoughts and how they affect my body. I am so thankful for my period and my body now and have so much more respect and love for them • during my two years of miscarriages a good friend gave me a book to read focusing on periods as a sacred pattern. My acupuncturist suggested extra rest. It had never occurred to me that my periods could deserve attention or consideration. I'm much happier now that I track and honour them • I rest when I need it. Qi gong therapy worked wonders for me some years ago and significantly reduced heavy flow, PMS and cramps. Young girls need to be taught how to find help if their periods are difficult and how to honour their body • getting a Mood Diary in my early 20s helped me to engage and appreciate my periods more • for years I hated and was confused by my period, my reproductive system, and my body. In my early 20s I was on the Pill and was terrified of getting pregnant. In my 30s I was diagnosed with PCOS, struggled with weight and body image and anxiously struggling to get pregnant. When I began fertility treatment I had a beautiful realization – I was supposed to love and cherish my body and the processes it was capable of! I began acupuncture, limited dairy and sugar, increased organic and healthful eating and exercised regularly. I was able to conceive naturally and adored my pregnancy! Now I see the value of loving my body and honouring all of its beautiful abilities • to help with her teenage PMS symptoms, I gave my daughter a Vitamin B drink every day from when she was eleven to seventeen. She was an angel in comparison to my friend's teenagers and has since thanked me for doing this • having just done a menopause workshop I feel much excitement at the prospect of menopause and the phase of life after. It also educated me on the selfcare I need to be doing now •

On finding a silver lining

Endometriosis runs my life. I cannot work, it limits my social life and activities and is the main focus in everything I do. Previously I've had several years without any symptoms and actually felt good while menstruating. I'm hopeful that I'll be able to experience that again. I love knowing that my female body is a gift, despite the sufferings I have with this disease, and that my menstrual blood is a sacred, life-giving part of the circle of life • having PCOS and fertility problems has made me appreciate menstruation much more – it would be nice if women felt empowered by the amazing miracle that their body performs each month, rather than feeling ashamed or dirty or embarrassed • even though I have fibroids and heavy bleeding now there have been many times where I have loved having my period and the heightened creativity, insight and feelings of oneness that it bestows • I am working on minimising the pain and the heaviness with food, rest and yoga – this is a work in progress. I feel excited and curious about working with my period and it's a reflection of my overall health •

Women would like to see health care providers who …

Understood the importance of regular menstrual cycles and were more sensitive to women who do not menstruate regularly • understood that women do know their own bodies, so listen to your patients! • were doctors that aren't males in stuffed shirts that don't understand a holistic approach to women • were better educated about menstruation: a doctor told me when I was a teenager that my period pain would go away once I had children, now at 47 years old I am still spending money on tampons, pain relief and psych visits for PMS! • would give me the best information, not only hormone replacement therapy! • had more up to date info on how supplement scan help ease or heal the causes of pain and other issues • understood women suffer as a result of menstrual problems such as my undiagnosed endometriosis • knew about more intimate issues, like how to manage your sex life during menopause • knew more about menopause so they can give us current and up to date resources • understood that fibroid cysts and heavy bleeding can be the first indicator that things are going awry. I wish there was more counselling for women on how NOT to have their parts removed • had offered treatment much earlier in my life. What a different kind of life I could have had • had more awareness about endometriosis, PCOS and other reproductive illnesses. Girls should NOT grow up thinking or being told by doctors it's normal to have bad period pain •

On options and informed choice

It would be great to have supportive educated medical professionals who understood the neurological and biological changes that can happen cyclically and hormonally and not jump to a 'mental health' diagnosis • I wish our gynes were more informed and not drug dealers, and that they wouldn't reprimand us for NOT taking their drugs • precise, CONSISTENT advice from health professionals would really help • I wish I had known much earlier that periods don't have to be painful – something that you just have to put up with! That you can seek help, make dietary adjustments, use exercise techniques and natural therapies, and try contraceptive methods other than the Pill! • I had a lot of pain growing up and have recently gone to an acupuncturist who solved the problem – it would have been great to get that support years ago • My deepest concern currently is the way that young women are prescribed hormonal contraception without being fully explained the side effects and the effect that this medication will have on their cycles. In the UK, there is so much fear around teenage pregnancy that little thought it given beyond that when prescribing these drugs. Young women I meet later in life are angry that they were not fully informed • doctors are too quick to prescribe HRT for menopause and too quick to prescribe the Pill for teenagers. If these stages in life were viewed as normal rather than pathological this would change • it would have been great to have had a doctor who understood PMS and didn't just say, 'you are depressed and need to go on medication' • I trialled different ways to deal with menopausal symptomology and I've found relief with naturopathy •

On menstrual mental health impacts

I really loathe and despise the prevalent discourse around PMS and the suggestion that it is a mental pathology (DSM-V). It seems as though PMS is another flaw that keeps women somehow at a lower level than rational, non-cyclical men in the very patriarchal medical and mental health profession discourse • there isn't enough information, research or support for people who suffer PMDD, so people who have it mostly suffer in silence and shame. It's really awful • I suffered terrible PMS for many years since age fourteen and only managed to get rid of the pain when I worked on the molestation I suffered as a child. I can't stress more the link between sickness and trauma and the power of healing • no one tells you menopause can be really traumatic psychologically and that it can bring up old traumas you thought were healed. They just tell you get on with it • On discovering mental health benefits I just wish that I could ALWAYS feel as wonderful and powerful and happy as I do on the last day of my period. (Not just because it's over for the month, but because I just feel soooo good about being me ... got to be a hormonal thing, I think) • I've always felt that menstruation is something special, I couldn't explain why. I intuitively felt that I was different those days, that I wanted to have a pause, stay relaxed and watch romantic movies • learning to respect and work with my cycle rather than pushing myself through it has been one of the tools that has helped me to heal from depression • I want to feel the power of my stronger feelings during menstruation without being overcome by them • the more open we are with others and particularly our friends and children, the better. Not just the physical 'facts' but emotional honesty about all that menstruation brings • I think it helps girls mature quicker than boys, and in that regard we have the upper hand. When we first get our period, we might not be ready for it or want it, but we just have to be responsible for it and get on with it, so to speak. No one else can deal with it for us. That's a pretty big lesson to learn and boys aren't really forced to learn that so early. On a deeper level, I think it helps us understand our emotions earlier too. We can reflect on our emotions/behaviours and different stages in our cycle and connect them to specific reasons, e.g. 'Oh, I just got my period, no wonder I was feeling so emotional last week …'. I think it helps females become more aware of our own bodies and emotion and I see that as an advantage •

The 'men' in menstruation

On what's unhelpful from men

Comments like: 'PMS does not actually exist' • men should be less grossed out by periods and not make women feel uncomfortable • men need to be less squeamish about it – total turn off if a guy can't even talk about it. I found after giving birth I can discuss anything about my cycle • I would like to have lovers who are not turned off by my menses • please may I never again hear a man accuse my bad mood on my period • my mum was a nurse and dad was a chiropractor and we were all brought up with it being a natural thing. When I got married I couldn't understand why my (then) husband treated me as an outcast during menstruation • my symptoms were so extreme that it was impossible to hide them from my father who decided that I willed it on myself. He eventually realised this was not the case • it began by being shamed and ridiculed by my father. I suffered from very severe PMS most of my life and kept it a very private matter with gradually less shame as I got older • when I was experiencing menopause I was married to a man who was very selfish, he gave me no support and my stress level was very high, the depression was the worst •

On the power of men who understand

A male Reiki teacher suggested I consider my period in a positive light. I now feel more connected to it and its purpose • how our men treat us during our bleed makes a big difference. If we're treated with affection and tenderness it goes a long way to help us accept and love ourselves • my husband has no problem picking up supplies, although a few times women have gotten snippy with him for even being in THAT aisle! Grow up, people! Many women have sympathised with him and have tried to help him select the proper pads. More power to them! • my husband is really understanding. He buys the stuff I need and does not bat an eyelid. Some husbands think it's a big deal if they buy some tampons, but he just acts normal and wants to help • I love the feeling of acceptance of my womanhood that making love during my period brings. This recently occurred with my partner after many years of misunderstanding about it, and a secret longing all that time • my husband is very open in talking about menstruation, which is fantastic • having a man who understands and acknowledges these life stages as normal and with whom I can talk about menopause has made all the difference • when I had my first period, my father brought me a rose. I was a bit embarrassed at the time, but also proud. Now it's a meaningful story I like to share • the men in my family were well educated about menstruation and were sensitive to women's issues. Perhaps they knew more than they wanted to know initially, but I believe it helped my brothers be more compassionate, understanding, supportive, and sensitive to girlfriends, wives, and daughters as well as moms and sisters • I was lucky enough to have a very open relationship with my dad and in fact he was the first person I told the morning I found I had my first period. I think it's important for dads to be involved, not just mums • it is interesting to note the diverse attitudes to periods of different partners I've had over time: from 'untouchable' to 'very sexy' • my husband was my hero throughout menopause. He made it safe for me to go into the hell and come back out safely • my menopausal libido is awful, and fatigue and fluctuations just overwhelm me sometimes. Thank God for a supportive husband! Ideas about education for boys and men I wish parents would teach their boys more and help them be more comfortable talking about it • I would like more men to understand it is a time for a woman to rest, reflect and to pamper herself • if women would speak openly with each other and with their male partners and friends, men would gain a deeper understanding • men and boys need more education not just about their own bodies, but about women's as well • I would like to see menstruation and menopause discussed openly and across genders • I wish men would have more education about it, as some are disgusted, and when I had partners like this it felt so maddeningly unfair • the more that I dive into menstrual awareness for myself the more that I am moved to honour the masculine and help men find their true power also. Women – and men too! – need to be taught from the start about the importance of the female's natural cycle, to celebrate and honour this, and to adapt life to work around the female cycle, rather than it being viewed as an inconvenience to have to deal with • men need to be taught about menopause too and how to support us. Hot flushes are invisible in the media – films and soap operas don't seem to feature women who have these. There is a spiritual element to it too. I think we need to speak about coming into our wisdom and the third age of woman. Embrace the validity of the older 'infertile' woman and help her regain her strength and value in society • I believe we need to inform men about how to be more sensitive to their partners during these major times of change in a woman's life • I know menopause is a powerful time but I don't think as a society we support the transition for most women. Men also need to be better educated about the process • I like being a crone. I found the rollercoaster of hormones unsettling. Great not having my husband comment anymore on my premenstrual/post-menstrual or any other tension • I feel too young for menopause. All my friends are very sexual beings still and I have ZERO sex drive yet am fit and thin, eat well and am healthy so I feel a little ripped off. My husband is in denial • I believe we need to inform men about how to be more sensitive to their partners during these major times of change in a woman's life •

Women's ideas about reframing menstruation and menopause

On reclaiming the menstrual cycle

Reclaiming my menstrual cycle has given me so much understanding about being a woman and being in the world. By using cloth pads and a Mooncup my connection with my blood and nature has deepened • every area of my life has benefitted by celebrating my bleeding time as a blessing. I am now approaching menopause and am finding ways to celebrate that too. My daughter is seven, but I already see how differently she feels about her body because I'm open and encouraging • it's my monthly rhythm, I use the energy I gain each time I bleed to feed my soul's growth • after having children I realised menstruation is such a wonderful gift • I have honoured my bleeding time in recent years and know how positively this affects my whole being • I enjoy examining the blood for signs of good health • I have always loved my bleeding and felt it was a privilege and honour, an intimate participation in the creative power of the universe • women are not encouraged to be messy. I finally felt liberated from the feeling of 'dirt' around my blood when I played with it – rubbed it into my body like war paint. Ironically I felt like a real woman rather than the 'china doll' version that old-fashioned values encourage • it is a very beautiful, wonderful, joyous, difficult thing to be a woman, but I treasure my femininity; it has made my life a wonder • despite the difficulties with my period, I have treasured my cycle throughout my life as a source of deep feminine wisdom, as one of the many rhythms of nature that bring to life a 'terrible beauty' • since learning about the cycles, tuning into the moon and embracing women's mysteries, I feel very grateful to be a woman and to have a period • I rejoice in my womb's transformational ability and feel lucky to be a woman who can have this physical connection to the earth's rhythms • how you feel about your period effects how you feel and experience significant events like giving birth and menopause. It's really important! • I honour my cycles they gave me my children • I have been exploring my cycle and its emotional/spiritual aspects for a few years and want to gain as much info and wisdom from this study as I can before I finish • I'm very grateful to be a cyclic woman. I love the seasons of my month and cherish the opportunities, physically, emotionally and spiritually, that my monthly cycle brings me • I have polycystic ovaries, and don't ovulate regularly, so when I do have a period I feel empowered, blessed and glad my body is working normally! • I enjoy the rhythm it gives my life and explore using different times of the cycle to advantage • I anticipate and welcome my bleeding. It's an opportunity to honour, withdraw and be gentle with myself. It's an important part of my identity • it's a great chance to cleanse and have a day of peace • I chart my cycle so know when I am due to bleed. The week before is an opportunity to release and let go emotionally, spiritually and physically. When I bleed, I feel deeply connected to the earth and my body, part of creation, strong and powerful I feel deeply reflective and go into myself for nourishment and contemplation • love the feeling of the blood flow, I love being a woman • before my period, I go through a reflective moment where I work out what I need to change in my life • menstruation is a very spiritual experience for me, I feel connected to my body and the rhythm of nature • I am now friends with my bleeds and every cycle I work towards healing and dropping the shame I have carried • since having two children I have learnt to honour this time and take it easy. It feels earthy and special and reminds me of where we all came from • it's my private time to unwind and be creative though I cannot have it all to myself since I'm a single mum and work full-time • fabulous and empowering – it is my daily compass •feel as if I'm releasing the old and starting afresh. It reminds me that I'm a woman and challenges me to embrace that and allow myself to be more vulnerable. It's a reminder of the strength I possess, the power to create, and to be gentle with myself because my body is hard at work. So many life lessons can be explored through the period • I relish the non-sexual, inward time and space • I appreciate how I am part of the earth, moon and cycles. Even if I know that being a mother is not for me I appreciate my body's ability to create life, and the life-giving capacity of my mind also • I have had thyroid problems and a regular cycle is a wonderful sign of health. I love getting it now! I feel feminine, powerful and validated • I feel the most connected to the land when I'm menstruating – earthy, centred and grounded • I am totally at peace with it, after having learned so much about it • I look forward to it each month. It reminds me of the life cycle and somehow grounds me and feels sacred • I feel blessed to have a healthy functioning body that has cyclical wisdom • my cycle is a gift and a reminder to slow down and rest • in my twenties I began to understand my rhythms better and now have had many years of creative, powerful cycles • I enjoy feeling more intuitive around my period. I especially enjoy the feminine power of the ability to help make and nurture another life! • I love it. I allow myself time to go dreamy and have a rest, at least some of the time. I don't do so much cooking for the family, I honour my blood, I have re-useable pads in gorgeous colours and pour my blood water on to the plants while I sing • I'm much more accepting of it now. I've had time to sort out my feelings, and actually, I find it rather magical! • I love it – I love the blood, I feel like a woman, I love the state of mind. I love that it is a doorway through which I can work with my boyfriend on our relationship and that I can touch base with myself • once the flow begins I let go, it's renewal and death in the same moment and one of the favourite parts of my life. The end is a feeling of completion, I feel at peace and realigned •

On the value of connecting with women over periods

I like bonding with other women in 'emergency' pad or tampon situations • I have been part of an online forum and we have a thread talking about our menstruation experiences. It's been a really supportive and beneficial group • compared to me my daughter and her friends have always been more open and she feels free discussing it with anyone she needs to • I wish there was more of a culture of celebrating menarche. I did this with a group of friends, even though we were all in our late 20s and 30s and had had periods for a long time. It was a very special and positive thing to do • I love the connection I have with my women friends who embrace it like I do • although it's inconvenient, emotional and painful I'm more connected with my sisterhood and feminine spirituality, so it also feels strengthening and powerful • I decided to embrace my menstruation as an important healing for not having had children and 20 years of disappointment. I make my own pads, call it my moon cycles and celebrate through poetry, art or quiet time. I meditate on menstrual pain as the pain of all women. I mark my period on a moon calendar and share stories and creating with other women • I felt pretty alone in it. Then I found a women's group for older women who are all experiencing similar life events (death of spouse, empty nest, menopause). We meet once a month for an afternoon potluck. I think this helped me more than anything. We eat, chat and support one another •

On how we can change this together

I took a class called Anthropology of Gender and we talked a lot about menstruation ceremonies, fertility, and the concept of the 'Red Tent'. It was really profound to me that there was a time in every month in which women in these societies were allowed to commune and rest, make craft, tell stories, sing songs, and pass these along generations of women. Teaching young women about the sacred nature of menstruation, birth, and female community, is crucial to keeping future generations in touch with female power, as well as shaping attitudes about menstruation, body-image and self-worth • I would love tools to share and pay forward to promote confidence, kindness and acceptance around menstruation • I dream of a world where menstruation is normalised and honoured for the miraculous process it is, and respected for its biological and cultural challenges • put it out there. Talk about it. If more of us discussed these topics openly there would be a lot less secrecy and misinformation • I'd like women and girls to learn that it does not have to be hard, it does mean a cycle is happening, it means look after yourself and love yourself better and understand the gift of living in an ever-changing body • gees, just TALK girls! There's no need to be so secretive • it's important to honour the beginning and end of menstruation, as well as each monthly cycle. Rest, nutrition, self-care, and self-love are all important to have a graceful menstrual period • more people need to be open and talk about it and get over their feelings of awkwardness or shame. Women should understand how their bodies work, including the full menstrual cycle, and men should learn about it as well • it would be nice if people were more in tune with their bodies and allowed themselves to slow down when they bleed. Society does not support that. Let's change it! • surely the information and details about our bodies and their functions should be openly discussed and supported, not in the form of shared horror stories, or tatty out-of-date pamphlets but in studies, films, forums and workshops • we can learn a lot

APPENDIX TWO

from the positive valuation of menstrual cycle from other cultures (Japan, China, Navaho) and try to apply it in modern life • I would really like all women to become aware of 'Red Tents' and the beneficial impact that type of nurturing and community can have for women of all ages in all places • any effort to restore this time to a sacred and honourable place in all our lives is really important. Women and men both need to develop awareness, understanding and positivity about both menstruation and menopause • On how we can better introduce girls to periods I would like to find a way to celebrate my daughter's first blood with her when it arrives. I wish that was done for me • when my daughter started hers we celebrated by going to the movies and getting pedicures • held a 'period party' for my daughter with women in our family, with her favourite food and by sharing interesting facts about menarche. It was a genuinely nice evening, no one had experienced anything like it • I'll hold a menarche ceremony for my daughter when the time comes. It's a special time, a rite of passage, and I believe it is important to mark it in a positive way • I would like to celebrate my daughter's transition to womanhood and let her know that it is a special time • a small period kit with fresh underwear baby wipes and bag for soiled clothes would have been a good way to avoid embarrassment • periods should really be celebrated as a sign of powerful femininity • having a child has made me much more comfortable with all aspects of my body as a woman and I plan on being extremely positive about it with my daughter • I'm crocheting a menarche blanket for my nine-year-old, who isn't anywhere near getting her period but I love how it facilitates conversations and her knowing that we'll celebrate her menarche when it comes • my daughter, her grandmothers and myself attended a preparation for menarche workshop. When she started bleeding a few months later she was so happy to be welcomed into the sisterhood. How wonderful if this becomes the norm!! • I wish young women would feel more empowered by their biology instead of always feeling like it is a negative impact on their health. I think of how as a girl we called our periods 'our friend'. I know what that meant I felt that way because it felt like a cleansing process when it occurred – very healthy • organised wonderful Red Parties for my two daughters when they got their first period. I think we should do more to celebrate this event and for this to be more accepted in society. There should be at least a special card and special dinner that day • we're preparing for my eleven-year-old daughter to have her period. She's excited • I really wish grandmothers, mothers, sisters, aunts were teaching young girls that periods are a blessing, not shameful, and feeling physically and mentally different during your period is okay • my daughter just began her period, two things I found most challenging was she didn't tell me (hoping it would go away) and used the word 'gross'. When I realised and spoke to her about it she cried for an hour! Her main fear was that her father and I wouldn't love her as much, that we would see her differently. I think she was very reassured by our responses as during her period she was very tender towards us and we her. I was also impressed with how she handled the logistics of pads • I am working to change periods for my daughters, we're getting excited and already looking at colourful cloth pads to celebrate them growing up • I have an eleven year old daughter and am proactively trying to create a more positive experience for her saying, 'It's a beautiful thing, a cleansing thing, a special thing our bodies do' • I have a son and a daughter and both can fetch a pad from the pile if I yell out from the bathroom. My daughter was around four when she started asking where I wanted my soak water poured in the garden. She knows blood grows babies and herbs! •

On how we can celebrate menarche

A feminist colleague's daughter just got her period, they celebrated, and she felt really proud. I wish every girl could feel like that • when my daughter got her period, I sent her flowers. I was really happy for her • my five-year-old daughter jumped up and down in excitement when she found out that one day she would also have blood in the toilet just like mumma • to ensure that my own daughters didn't suffer ignorance or embarrassment – I have been very open with them. They were prepared with pads in their school bags in case it started at school. We went out for dinner, dressing in 'red' items to celebrate their womanhood when their periods did start. They loved that! • I wrote a book for my oldest granddaughter in order to make her first period a celebration, which we celebrated last year. It went over so well! • when my daughter got hers, I took her out to the movies and lunch to celebrate instead of the negative hush hush, it's something you don't talk about attitude. She is a lot more open and will tell her father, brother and male friends to leave her alone and why she is feeling upset • I think it is important that we educate young girls that the beginning and end of menstruation are rites of passage. Let's make them sacred events •

On attitudes to menopause and what would help

I think it's a shame that women tend to discuss menopause so little, fearing to mention their discomfort or aging, when it would help other women to share experiences and information • I know menopause is a powerful time, but I don't think as a society we support the transition for most women. Men also need to be better educated about the process •

On recommendations for reframing menopause

We need to completely re-think menopause. We can help ourselves by listening to our intuition, to our bodies, possibly changing our diets, our habits and patterns, using herbs and other natural non-invasive remedies to minimise difficult symptoms. We now have a wealth of information to help us to make positive decisions about what is best for us as individuals. We need to accept that we are growing older with equanimity, at the very least, if not excitement! • I remember with delight the stage show Menopause the Musical, wonderful cartoons from Judy Horacek and others that have enabled us to speak openly and proudly about our bodies and changes. Thank you, brave sisters, • menopause is a natural progression in a woman's life and, contrary to ads, we do not turn into dried up old women with humps on our back! • menopause is a celebration of becoming a wise and beautiful older woman, something I am enjoying • women's bodies are beautiful and still somewhat a mystery. We need to 'normalise' all aspects of a woman's life span • healing, compassion and liberation are also side-effects of menopause. Finding our authentic selves, our real voices, our heart's desires, freed from the lovely tyranny of hormones, we can step into the next phase with power and purpose, love, compassion and deep joy. YAY!!!! The world so needs us!! • I would like to see older women actively honoured in their role as crones – the wise women of the tribe – and heaps more work needs to be done to celebrate these important times of transition/rites of passage • I experienced an intense spiritual awakening during both puberty and menopause like I have never experienced at any other time in my life • I would like there to be less shame and embarrassment associated with menstruation and menopause. I want them to be seen as powerful and creative processes that celebrate me as a woman • let's see positive representations of menopause in the media • recent ads that celebrate womanhood in all its phases are a delight • talk to your girlfriends and read, read, read. There are some really good books out there • I would like to see menopause honoured as more part of life rather than something that has to be hidden and not discussed • I likened peri-menopause to the last trimester of pregnancy, only instead of a baby being born, I WAS BORN, me the grown-up WOMAN •

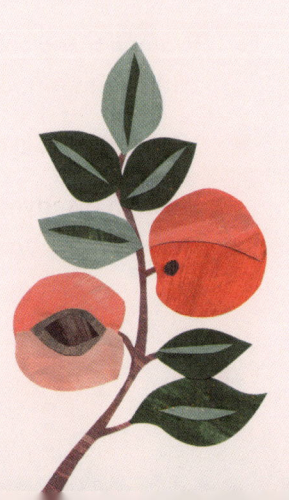

Appendix Three: Menstrual Shame

Brené Brown's articulation of shame in her book *I Thought It Was Just me (But It Isn't)* is valuable in helping us to understand menstrual shame, and most importantly how to develop resilience to it.

Brené Brown makes a clear distinction between embarrassment, humiliation, guilt and shame. While these are all clearly related, and may move from one to another, even overlapping, the primary difference between them is this:

- Embarrassment is the least powerful, and may later lead to laughter at our own folly

- Humiliation is a form of belittlement by another

- Guilt is when we do something we know is wrong. I did it, but I can change my behaviour and may be able to right the wrong by taking responsibility and atoning

- Shame is an internalised message. It becomes who we are

- Guilt – I have done wrong. Shame – I am wrong.

Using Brown's modelling of shame to look specifically at the kind of shame produced and maintained by the menstrual taboo we can see that menstrual shame has resulted in:

- Lack of understanding of the menstrual cycle

- Absence of a model of menstrual wellbeing and how to achieve and maintain it

- Few social and cultural environments conducive to menstrual wellbeing

- Women being vulnerable to 'expert' recommendations to eliminate ovulation / menstruation without informed choice or even knowing it's happening

- Women not seeking or receiving adequate health care for menstrual problems

- Women disadvantaged in various ways through the abnormalisation of menstruation and menstruating bodies

APPENDIX THREE

- Emotional and physical harm from the direct experience of embarrassment, humiliation and shame regarding menstruation.

So how do we develop resilience to shame, and specifically menstrual shame?

According to Brené Brown shame diminishes our capacity for empathy, because if we believe in some innate inadequacy in ourselves we can certainly believe it of others. But it also uses precious emotional resources in a harmful and destructive pursuit. Shame has no momentum or onus for action. But as Brown argues, we all have shame and we are all captive to it at different points in our lives. Many of our social constructs (religion, capitalism, relationships) use shame to incapacitate and control people. So we need to build up ways of coping with it, and strategies to break its power over us. Brown calls this shame resilience and it's very helpful for us to consider how she approaches the building of it.

Firstly, she explains, it's vital to recognise the personal vulnerability that led to the feelings of shame, or accepting that you are a person with emotions and triggers, who will likely feel shame over certain things due to your background and experiences. The next step, of crucial importance to us in deconstructing menstrual shame, is to examine and acknowledge the external factors that led to the feelings of shame, or the things that are bigger than you and out of your experience and control. This is why we have looked at the menstrual taboo, throughout history and across cultures, so we can see that our own experiences are not the only influence on how we view menstruation and the stigma often associated with it.

Next, Brown counsels that connecting with others to receive and offer empathy is a powerful antidote to shame, for all participating. And finally, discussing and deconstructing the feelings of shame themselves, so that we can see them for what they are, and lessen the power they have to hold us back.

Shame resilience requires the courage to tell our stories and compassion to hear the shame of others, as well as a critical approach where we look at the big picture outside of our own personal lives.

Appendix Four: The Victorian Women's Trust Menstrual and Menopause Wellbeing Policy

Rationale

Experiences of menstruation and menopause can be very debilitating, yet we have been enculturated to mask their existence in the workplace, at schools and at home. This policy supports employees in their ability to adequately self-care during their period and menopause, while not being penalised by having to deplete their sick leave. Periods and menopause are not a sickness after all. This policy also seeks to remove the stigma and taboo surrounding menstruation and menopause.

A recent VWT survey of 3,460 people in Australia and around the world showed that:

- 58 per cent of respondents who have experienced menstruation said that a day off to rest would make their period a better experience every month.

- 26 per cent of those who had gone through menopause said that being able to take time off when needed would have helped their transition.

- 24 per cent of those surveyed said that being able to ask for what they need from their employer would make their period a better experience.

Policy

This policy is designed to provide opportunities for restful working circumstances and self-care for employees experiencing symptoms of menstruation and menopause.

The policy is designed to be flexible depending on the employee's needs, providing for the following options:

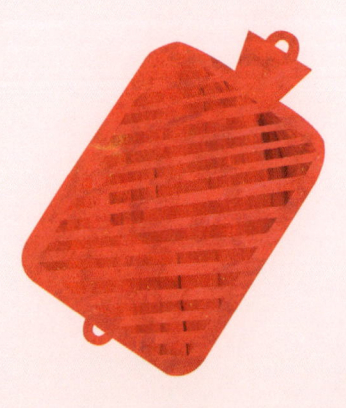

1. The possibility of working from home;

2. The opportunity to stay in the workplace under circumstances which encourage the comfort of the employee eg. resting in a quiet area; or

3. The possibility of taking a day's paid leave.

In the case of paid leave, employees are entitled to a maximum of 12 paid days per calendar year (pro-rata, non-cumulative) in the event of inability to perform work duties because of menstruation and menopause, and their associated symptoms.

A medical certificate is not required.

Staff needing to use this policy must contact the Executive Director and indicate which options they will be taking on the day.

Length of allowance

The Victorian Women's Trust's entitlement of up to 12 paid days a year would be in line with the national and international standards.

References and Notes

Authors' Note

i   **Trans:** abbreviation of transgender or transgenderism, used as an adjective relating to transition between assigned genders, from the Latin meaning 'across from', or 'on the other side of'.

   Cis: abbreviation of cisgender, a term developed in the 1990s to describe people whose gender identity conforms to the sex they were assigned at birth, from the Latin meaning 'on this side of'.

   Gender non-conforming: another adjective relating to people who do not identify as either binary gender (male or female). Related terms include gender diverse, genderqueer, and gender non-binary.

Introduction

i   Bennett, J & Pope, A 2008, *The Pill: Are You Sure It's for You?*, Sally Milner Publishing, Bowral, p.202.

The Biological Integrity of Menstruation

i   wikipedia.org/wiki/Sexual_differentiation, has more on these conditions.

ii While this is the generally accepted wisdom there is some evidence emerging from research into mice that suggests that mammals may be able to produce new egg cells during their fertile years if the ovary is damaged: another case of watch and see. See Zou, K. et al., 2009, 'Production of offspring from a germline stem cell line derived from neonatal ovaries', *Nature Cell Biology*, vol. 11, iss. 5, pp. 631-6.

iii The clitoris continues to grow throughout a woman's life, rather like ears and noses do. No age-related atrophy there!

iv Note on these statistics: the age group numbers were averaged, but this is not an overall average of all women, and the numbers in each age group differ.

REFERENCES AND NOTES

v Mark Hanson and Peter Gluckman respectively head the Centre for the Developmental Origins of Health and Disease (DOHaD) at the University of Southampton (UK), and the Liggins Institute at the University of Auckland (NZ) liv Hanson, M & Gluckman, P 2005, 'New research shows how evolution explains age of puberty' *ScienceDaily*, <www.sciencedaily.com/releases/2005/12/051201022811.htm>.

vi Interestingly, the hypothalamus and the pituitary gland are responsive to increased levels of light, such as that of the full moon, so perhaps it's no accident that our cycles are generally (lunar) monthly. Research in the 1950s and 60s by Dr Eugene Jonas and his colleagues found a significant link between fertility and the lunar cycle, particularly heightened potential for ovulation at the return of the angle between the sun and moon (which happens monthly) that was present at a woman's birth. At the time there was a flurry of interest on both sides of the Atlantic and numerous papers on it published in medical journals until the Pill was approved and promised greater simplicity for doctors, patients and accountants. See Naish. F, 2004, *Natural Fertility: the Complete Guide to Avoiding or Achieving Conception*, Sally Milner Publishing, Australia.

vii The 28-day cycle of the Pill is not a menstrual cycle as ovulation is almost always suppressed and the 'period' is a withdrawal bleed triggered by the start of the seven days of placebo pills.

viii Lin, J 2011, 'Plasticity of human menstrual blood stem cells derived from the endometrium', *Journal of Zhejiang University*, May, vol.12, iss. 5, pp.372–380, <www.ncbi.nlm.nih.gov/pmc/articles/PMC3087093/>

ix Miller, G et.al. 2007, 'Ovulatory cycle effects on tip earnings by lap dancers: economic evidence for human estrus?', *Evolution and Human Behavior*, vol. 28, pp. 375-381.

x See www.menstruationresearch.org for examples

xi Billings, E 1980, *The Billings Method*, Penguin, Australia, p.13.

xii ibid.

xiii Stepanich-Reidling, KK 1992, *Sister Moon Lodge: the Power and Mystery of Menstruation*, Llewellyn Worldwide.

xiv Brown, J 1980, 'The scientific basis of the Ovulation Method', in Billings, J.J. et.al., *The Billings Atlas of the Ovulation Method*, Ovulation Method Research and Reference Centre of Australia.

xv Kaminsky, L 2018, 'The case for renaming women's body parts', <http://www.bbc.com/future/story/20180531-how-womens-body-parts-have-been-named-after-men>.

xvi Kellermeier, K, *How Menstruation Created Mathematics*, <http://faculty.plattsburgh.edu/john.kellermeier/Menses/Menses.htm>.

xvii Darling, D 2004, *The Universal Book of Mathematics: From Abracadabra to Zeno's Paradoxes*, Turner Publishing Company, Hoboken.

xviii Grahn, J, 1993, *Blood Bread and Roses: How Menstruation Created the World*, Beacon Press, Massachusetts, p. xi.

xix Emera, D, Romero, R And Wagner, G 2011, The evolution of menstruation: A new model for genetic assimilation: Explaining molecular origins of maternal responses to fetal invasiveness, *BIOESSAYS*, 7 November.

xx Northrup, C 2012, *The Wisdom of Menopause (Revised Edition): Creating Physical and Emotional Health During the Change*, Random House, New York.

xxi Hrdy, SB 2000, *Mother Nature*, Ballantine Books, p.102.

xxii Pearce, LH 2012, *Moon Time: Harness the Ever-Changing Energy of Your Menstrual Cycle*, Womancraft Publishing, Cork.

xxiii Hrdy, SB 2000, *Mother Nature*, Ballantine Books, p.102.

xxiv Ibid., p.102.

xxv Ibid., p.282

A Pervasive Menstrual Taboo

i Fershtman, C, Gneezy, U & Hoffman, M 2011, 'Taboos and Identity: considering the unthinkable', *American Economic Journal: Microeconomics*, vol. 3, no. 2, pp. 139-164.

ii Witt, C & Shapiro, L, 2018 'Feminist history of philosophy', *The Stanford Encyclopedia of Philosophy*, (Fall edition), Zalta EN (ed.), URL <http://plato.stanford.edu/archives/fall2018/entries/feminism-femhist/>.

iii Hall, N, Barbosa, MC, Currie, D, Dean, AJ, Head, B, Hill, PS, Naylor, S, Reid, S, Selvey, L and Willis, J 2017, Water, sanitation and hygiene in remote Indigenous Australian communities: A scan of priorities', *Global Change Institute discussion paper: Water for equity and wellbeing series*, The University of Queensland, Brisbane.

iv McCormack, A 2017, 'Free sanitary item vending machines installed in SA schools', *ABC Online*, 11 August, last accessed 23 May 2018, <https://www.abc.net.au/triplej/programs/hack/sanitary-vending-machines/8797764>.

v 'Progress on sanitation and drinking water: 2015 update and MDG assessment', UNICEF and World Health Organisation, <https://www.unicef.org/publications/index_82419.html>.

REFERENCES AND NOTES

vi   UNESCO, 'Good Policy and Practice in Health Education: Puberty Education and Menstrual Hygiene Management', 2014, <https://unesdoc.unesco.org/ark:/48223/pf0000226792>.

vii   A.C. Nielsen and Plan India, 2010, 'Sanitation protection: Every Women's Health Right. Goyal, also mentioned in Vishakha, 2016, 'Scope and opportunities for menstrual health and hygiene products in India', *International Research Journal of Social Sciences*, vol. 5, pp. 2319-3565.

viii   Bullman, M 2017, 'Girls from low-income families skipping school during periods because they can't afford sanitary products', 14 March, *The Independent*, United Kingdom.

ix   Schooler, D, Ward, LM, Merriwether, A & Caruthers, AS 2005, 'Cycles of shame: menstrual shame, body shame and sexual decision-making', *Journal of Sex Research*, November 2005.

x   Roberts, T & Waters, PL, 2008, 'Self-objectification and that "Not So Fresh Feeling": Feminist therapeutic interventions for healthy female embodiment', *Women and Therapy*, vol. 27, nos. 3-4, pp. 5-21.

xi   Gaslighting is a form of psychological manipulation that seeks to sow seeds of doubt in a targeted individual or members of a targeted group, making them question their own memory, perception and sanity. *Oxford English Dictionary*, retrieved from <www.oxforddictionaries.com> 2019.

xii   Brown, B. 2008, *I Thought It Was Just Me (But It Isn't)*, Gotham Books, New York.

xiii   Lord, E 2017, 'After this woman's male co-worker period-shamed her, HR took his side', Bustle, 19 July, Last accessed 23 May 2018, <https://www.bustle.com/p/after-this-womans-male-co-worker-period-shamed-her-hr-took-his-side-71093>.

xiv   'ACLU appeals case of Georgia woman fired for getting her period at work' 2017, ACLU, Press Release, 17 August 2017, <https://www.aclu.org/news/aclu-appeals-case-georgia-woman-fired-getting-her-period-work> last accessed 23 May 2018.

xv   In private email dated 2016

xvi   Skovlund, CW, Morch, LS & Kessing, LV 2016, 'Association of Hormonal Contraception with Depression'. *JAMA Psychiatry*, 2016, vol.73, iss. 11, pp. 1154-1162.

xvii   Bennett, J and Pope, A 2008, *The Pill: Are You Sure It's For You?*, Allen and Unwin, Sydney.

xviii   Hoffman, DE & Tarzian, AJ, 2008 'The girl who cried pain: A bias against women in the treatment of pain', *The Journal of Law, Medicine and Ethics*, vol. 28 (sup 4), pp. 13-27.

xix   Ussher, JM & Perz, J 2013, 'PMS as a process of negotiation: women's experience and management of premenstrual distress', *Journal of Psychology and Health*, vol. 28, no. 8, pp. 909-27.

xx   American College of Obstetricians and Gynecologists, 2015, 'Menstruation in Girls and Adolescents: Using the Menstrual Cycle as a Vital Sign', Committee Opinion No. 651, December 2015 <https://www. acog.org/-/media/CommitteeOpinions/Committee-on-Adolescent-Health-Care/ co651.pdf?dmc=1&>.

xxi   Endometriosis Australia, last accessed 23 May 2018 <https://www.endometriosisaustralia.org/research>.

xxii   Jean Hailes for *Women's Health*, last accessed 23 May 2018, <https://jeanhailes.org.au/health-a-z/pcos>.

xxiii   Motluk, A 2007, 'Menstrual blood could be rich source of stem cells', *New Scientist*, 15 November, <https://www.newscientist.com/article/dn12924-menstrual-blood-could-be-rich-source-of-stem-cells/>.

xxiv   Centers for Disease Control (CDC), 1982, 'Toxic-shock syndrome, United States, 1970-1982', *Morbidity and Mortality Weekly Report*, 1982 Apr 30, vol. 31, iss. 16, pp201-4.

xxv   Edraki, F 2017, 'Tampons, pads, menstrual cups, period underwear: what's best for the environment?' *ABC Online*, 4 November, <http://www.abc.net.au/ news/2017-10-27/which-period-product-is-best-for-the-environment/9090658>.

xxvi   Brown, K & Gruber, I 2015, 'What on earth is a moon cup?' *Choice Magazine*, 27 October, <https://www.choice.com.au/health-and-body/reproductive-health/womens-health/ buying-guides/menstrual-cups>.

xxvii   Delaney, J, Lupton, MJ & Toth, E 1988, *The Curse: A Cultural History of Menstruation*, First University of Illinois Press, Illinois.

xxviii   Patton, GC et al.,1996, 'Menarche and the onset of depression and anxiety in Victoria, Australia', *Journal of Epidemiology and Community Health*, Dec; vol. 50, iss. 6, pp. 661-6.

xxix   Baxter, B 2017, *Ending a Workplace Taboo. Period*, video recording, TEDxBristol, <https://www.youtube.com/watch?v=0wWUAx_1JDw>.

Dismantling the Menstrual Taboo

i   Plan International 2017, 'The Dream Gap: Australian Girls' View on Gender Equality', October, <https://apo.org.au/sites/default/files/resource-files/2017/10/apo-nid113711-1232136.pdf>